To Sam Perry

much Love
Susixxx

BE
FREE

A Holistic Guide to Freedom from Anxiety,
Stress and Low Mood for Life

Susi McWilliam

BALBOA
PRESS
A DIVISION OF HAY HOUSE

Balboa Press books may be ordered through booksellers or by contacting:

Balboa Press
A Division of Hay House
1663 Liberty Drive
Bloomington, IN 47403
www.balboapress.co.uk
1 (877) 407-4847

Print information available on the last page.

ISBN: 978-1-9822-8076-5 (sc)
ISBN: 978-1-9822-8074-1 (hc)
ISBN: 978-1-9822-8075-8 (e)

Balboa Press rev. date: 06/14/2019

To my late mother, Jenny, the kindest, most compassionate person I've ever known and my biggest cheerleader and inspiration. I did it, Mum.

ACKNOWLEDGEMENTS

Thank you to my family. My husband, Stuart, supported me when I was bedridden and as I followed my dream to create this book to help others. Thanks also to my amazing children, Erin, Cammie, and Lili, who drive me to be the best mother and role model I can be.

I also want to thank the best mother, my mum, Jenny. Sadly, she's no longer on this earth, but I know she is still supporting me, loving me, and guiding me. She drives me forward when I think I cannot manage. I also thank my sister, brother, and dad, for family is my safe place.

To my best friend, Erika Cowie, who has held my hand through life and through this creation; she's my anchor, rock, and sounding board.

To my coach and friend, Calea Souter, who allowed me to see my capabilities, helped me deal with being overwhelmed, and pushed me to submit the book, despite rejections.

To my spiritual teachers who have guided me along the way: Zoe Toussaint-Winchcombe, Karina Stewart, Louise Hay, Gabrielle Bernstein, Rebecca Campbell, and other Hay House authors.

Thank you to all my amazing clients over the years; they taught me so much about anxiety, depression, and stress, and they also taught me about myself. Thanks for the friendships we've made and the journey we shared together. You are my inspiration.

Contents

DISCLAIMER

This book is not intended as a substitute for medical advice from doctors. Readers should consult a doctor on all matters relating to their health and in particular with respect to any symptoms that may require medical attention. Seek appropriate professional and medical support when necessary.

How to Use This Book

This book has been created to give you the tools to overcome anxiety, reduce stress, and improve mood. It's a guidebook back to being free, to help you move forward and live the life you deserve. You can dip in and out if you're feeling particularly stressed or overwhelmed, or you can work through the whole book, step by step, embracing it all and completely ramping up your lifestyle.

It will get easier.

I created the Be Free Anxiety Matrix after realising that overcoming anxiety couldn't be achieved by one single action or solution. As I spent my time looking for solutions and studying results, the matrix came to fruition. The matrix is the base for my anxiety coaching work.

BE FREE: ANXIETY MATRIX
by Spirit and Soul

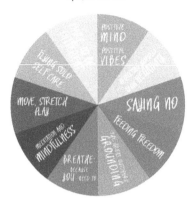

It is this holistic view that gives results that last forever. Dr Benjamin Snider, a naturopathic doctor, said, "It's critical that you're not just looking at the physical causes, because if you are experiencing anxiety the single causative factor may exist in the beliefs you hold about yourself, or it might exist in unresolved emotional conflict from your past. Many times, the body will express anxiety as a way of discharging anxiety felt earlier in your life. The body's way of healing." The matrix and the areas covered within it offer an opportunity to review a number of areas of your life which maybe be leading to your anxiety

You may have already explored some areas and ideas; that's fabulous. You'll be off to a flying start. Revisiting these ideas will give you the opportunity to reignite and inspire you to explore solutions further.

If you haven't heard of these things, then why not try introducing some new ideas, exercises, and activities? It's time for change.

Take your time; implement changes step by step. Small changes will lead to big changes. Maybe take one exercise and do it for a week, and then add another. It is a gradual process. Know that every step you take will have you feeling more vibrant and healthier in your mind, body, and soul. You will radiate this vibrancy out to those around you and to the world. You'll begin to get your life back. Step by step, you will feel more confident, empowered, and more like you. You'll feel better than you ever have before, fully present and fully you, leading the life you deserve.

The focus is to build in habits that will last. If you find yourself getting overwhelmed at any point, take a step back and then revisit it later.

Keep a journal or diary as you read through this book, or make notes inside it. It's a great tool to look back at on the days when you feel low. I guarantee you will be making progress every day without even realising it.

At the beginning of each chapter, you will be given an affirmation: a positive statement to repeat as many times as you can throughout the day, especially if you are feeling a bit low or overwhelmed. These little words will help support you, guide you, and show you just how amazing you truly are.

Whether you suffer from generalised anxiety, panic disorder, social anxiety, or low mood, or are feeling super overwhelmed and stressed, these exercises and ideas will help guide, support, inspire, and lead you to your life of freedom.

Be free.
Love and live your light,
Susi
xxxxxx

My Story

Struggling with anxiety, low mood, panic, and stress? What if there were a solution, a magical cure so that no matter what life threw at you, you would be able to cope better? Would you be willing to do what it takes to create peace in your life?

When I was 15, I started suffering from panic attacks. These started when I was out with friends, and there seemed to be no rhyme or reason to their happening. The more that they happened, the faster they came. In the doctor's office with my mum, I was prescribed beta blockers and antidepressants. It's strange; even at 15, although I knew in my head I'd been offered a solution, it didn't sit right with me. I wanted to know why the panic attacks were happening. I didn't want to take man-made drugs. Anyway, I carried on and never took them. I attended yoga with my mum, tried homeopathy and hypnotherapy, and looked at alternative support. Fast-forward another couple of years, and then I started drinking. The panic attacks would worsen the self-loathing, and then when drunk, I would hate myself so much I would self-harm. I would despise myself, which led to me punching and slapping myself. Whilst all this was going on, I would be the life and soul of the party, and I had great friends, the most amazing family, and a wonderful life. This fuelled my guilt and upset me more. What right did I have to feel low or down when others had it so much worse?

A few years later, I started uni, bought a flat, and worked, always super motivated and wanting to find the key to happiness. I did everything to excess. I studied, partied, and worked two jobs. It was fun, but my body kept trying to tell me otherwise. I had more panic attacks, psoriasis over my whole body, and a gripping in my chest.

After university, I tried different jobs. I had my own catering business, which I worked from the early mornings late into the night, and continued to party. Relationships started to fall apart; the stress grew too much. Whilst on a holiday with friends, I decided enough was enough and said I wasn't coming home. I decided to run, run away from my life and responsibilities. Whilst making this decision, I hurt those I loved most: my family. The guilt of my leaving them worried and concerned was too much, and I flew home to face the music. As you can imagine, this fuelled my self-loathing and anxiety even more. I felt trapped, lost, and a failure.

By my late twenties, I was getting on well with work, successful, with a lovely flat and new boyfriend (now my husband)—everything was going well. I still had the occasional panic attack, but I was now becoming more aware and in tune with triggers and with things that were supporting me and helping me feel better.

I always placed a lot of pressure on myself to be the best at what I did, always giving 110 per cent. After marrying Stuart, I became a stepmum to two children. I focused all my attention on being the best wife to my husband and the best support for the children. I loved children dearly and had always wanted a big family. We then started trying for our own baby, only to be told that we were not going to be able to conceive a child together naturally. Despite everything I've mentioned above, I kept pushing, kept driving, and was motivated. I was unwilling to accept that was the case. I figured there must be a natural solution. Again, I gave 110 per cent into looking at diets, nutrition, acupuncture, and positions. Then the magic happened. Call it a miracle or that we'd successfully managed to improve our health, but we had a little baby girl.

I was delighted but quite naive as to the stress and pressure I was going to endure. It wasn't an easy pregnancy health-wise, made even more difficult by the dynamics of not having a typical nuclear family. It was tough. Once my beautiful girl was here, I started to experience all sorts of health concerns: panic attacks and feeling like I was going to black out, and then I got labyrinthitis and BPPV, an inner ear condition which affected my balance.

My world started to get smaller. This condition would disappear and then reoccur. I would be driving with the kids and suddenly feel like I was going to pass out. The anxiety I was feeling was off the scale. I had a constant tightness in my chest. I'd convinced myself I had a brain tumour or was going to have a heart attack.

I went to the hospital, and they diagnosed me with subconscious hyperventilation and postnatal depression. In my usual style and response, I disagreed. I looked again for natural solutions and found an amazing natural medicine practitioner. I turned up with my list of symptoms. She reviewed these, my history from birth, and my diet. She diagnosed adrenal fatigue, which is caused by living in a state of stress. She implemented some solutions and changed my diet, and within a couple of weeks, I felt so much better. It was another miracle, as far as I was concerned.

Feeling better and living my life, the next curveball hit. I was lying on the sofa one night, and then I had severe pain in my abdomen. It was excruciating. I then started to bleed from down below. I called the medical helpline, as it was a Friday night, and they made an appointment for me to see a doctor straight away. This doctor told me that it would pass and it was probably something I'd eaten and my time of the month. Yet again, I was losing confidence in the medical profession. I was so upset. I don't know why, but in that moment, I drove to a local supermarket and bought a pregnancy test. It tested positive. I bought three more, and they were all the same. I was so excited yet terrified. I continued testing the next two days, with the lines getting fainter. I visited my GP on the Monday to be told it had been an early miscarriage. I was devastated. I blamed myself, although I hadn't even known. It really fuelled everything I'd been battling and burying deep down.

We spoke to medical professionals again to see if we could have another baby. They told us it was impossible for us to conceive again but that we could try in vitro fertilization. I couldn't get my head around it all.

We started the IVF process, and my heart and head were all over the place. My controlling nature was kicking in, telling me that I could achieve anything I wanted and wouldn't stop until I got it. We were taught how to give injections and everything that was involved; I had my ovaries checked. As I sat in a room of other hopeful would-be parents at the hospital, I realised I couldn't do it to myself. Mentally, I couldn't cope with another miscarriage or with the hormonal changes. My egg-removal appointment was booked, and I bailed.

I felt like a failure that I didn't have the strength to continue. The panic attacks had kicked in full scale, and I was struggling to get my daughter from the nursery, go out for dinner, and do the things I loved. I went to my GP again and asked for antidepressants. I cried as I picked up my prescription and popped that little pill into my mouth. I started to read the side effects and completely freaked myself out. I had a panic attack and again ended up on the phone to the doctors. I knew then I wouldn't take any more. I fell into a complete breakdown.

For days, I lay in bed, unable to get up and cope. I was numb. My body gave up and shut down. I felt no emotion. I couldn't eat. I lay in bed and watched TV, unaware even of what I was watching. Stuart was left to look after the children, along with my mum. They tried to buy me foods I liked and feed me nutritious food, but I was switched off to the world, switched off to my children. I slowly started to awaken, to realise that what I wanted most in the world was to be there for my kids, not to be a zombie.

As I lay in bed, I started to look back at things that had helped me previously. I loved meditation as a teen in my yoga classes, so I started listening to meditations whilst in bed on a loop. A friend advised me to try reiki, and that changed my world. It opened me up to why I was doing what I was doing and how to improve my life, then it grew and expanded. Each day or week, I would add something else to the mix to help me find peace, happiness, and health. I researched constantly, trying new things and natural health solutions. I studied nutrition, crystals, and oils and discovered self-care.

That is where this book was born. I've found natural solutions that can truly allow you to take your life back. Everything in this book has been tried and tested and used by me. The day I decided to look for solutions has now led me on a beautiful and challenging journey to where I'm at today. I am now a holistic health and anxiety coach, qualified reiki practitioner, meditation teacher to adults and children, and essential oil enthusiast. My goal is to share and empower others to find solutions to their anxiety, stress, and ill health.

I hope that this book helps you discover your own journey to peace and happiness. It's only a decision away. You've got this.

Love and live your light.

Susi

xxxxx

CHAPTER 1
Positive Mind, Positive Vibes:
Reprogramming your Mindset for Freedom

> I choose only loving words and positive
> thoughts, and my mind thanks me for it.

Brain Training (Programming your brain) may be something you associate with a Nintendo DS game or something you may have done at school. Not something you'd do to help get you onto a path of peace, calm, and tranquillity. Sounds like hard work, huh?

Guess what? It is a little bit of work, but not hard work. This is an area I am hugely passionate about, and that's why I'm covering it first. Because without it, regardless of what you eat, how much exercise you take, or however many treatments you try, you will never be free from anxiety, stress, and low mood.

Once you start working with your mind and your thoughts, your whole world will change. I truly believe that from the bottom of my heart. I'll tell you why. As

I lay in my bed, ill with my room spinning, imagining I was never going to get better, that panic attacks and feeling like I might die would be a constant in my life, I made a decision. Because I couldn't read or watch TV without feeling awful, I would listen. I searched on YouTube, and this is where things started to change. I chose to listen to affirmations on a loop. I listened to affirmations and healing meditations every day. I didn't believe everything I heard, but I kept listening. During these periods of meditation and affirmations, I felt better. Somehow clearer and happier. I decided to wake each day, pick an affirmation, and repeat it and repeat it and repeat it. To this day, I meditate and use affirmations daily.

Not sure what an affirmation is? An affirmation is a positive saying or phrase about yourself. It provides emotional support and encouragement. Here are some examples:

My body is happy, healthy, and vibrant.
I am a positive and friendly person.
I make a positive contribution, and I am valued.
I am brave, fearless, and passionate.
I am awesome, amazing, fabulous, and so on.

Try it now; repeat the following: "I am awesome, amazing, and fabulous." How did that feel? Try it again. "I am awesome, amazing, and fabulous." Does it feel funny? Are you giggling, or does it make you feel really uncomfortable?

We're so used to hearing that negative chat in our heads that saying positive things about ourselves can feel a little uncomfortable.

What does the voice in your head tell you? Tune into it more, and if you're reading this book, it's probably not pleasant. Does it say, "Hey, you. Hey, beautiful, what a great job you did getting through that day. You rock!" Hmmmmmm. Mine certainly never used to. It said things like "You're so stupid! You seriously need to get a life. What a loser! You're overweight. Stop being such a freak. I can't believe you can't even go shopping without freaking out. Your husband will probably leave you. You're so boring ..." Seriously, it was out of control. But I believed it all, and my body and mind reacted accordingly.

It consumed me and swallowed me up. It bullied me, made me feel small, filled me with doubt, and fuelled my insecurities.

In the words of C. S. Lewis, "We are what we believe we are." This is not just a beautiful quote but a scientific fact. The brain responds the same way to a mental thought as it would if you carried out a physical task. So if you think about spiders, for example, and how much they scare you, your brain doesn't know the difference between you thinking about seeing a spider and being scared or actually seeing the spider. It will release the same stress hormones and responses whether it's real or imaginary.

As you can see, if we're constantly thinking about what ifs and focusing on the negative, it won't take long before our body is filled with stress hormones, such as cortisol, and responding in fight-or-flight mode, making us feel edgy, stressed, and anxious.

Fight-or-flight mode is the body's protective mechanism for coping with life-threatening or potentially dangerous situations. It's handy if you're running away from a sabretooth tiger in caveman times, but not so handy if it triggers just because you are late for a meeting or are away to do a talk. It's the body's way of preparing for an extremely stressful situation. This response can make your heart race, you might feel sweaty, your vision may narrow, you might need the loo, and even your hearing becomes more sensitive. It's not the best feeling in the world, and once it's passed, you can be left feeling drained and low. Negative thoughts narrow your mind and world.

So what can we do to help ourselves? It's not all doom and gloom. Just as our brain can't tell the difference between a negative thought and a negative experience, the same can be said for positive thoughts and experiences. Pretty cool. This blows my mind, and this is what will change your life. These techniques are used by top-level executives, NASA astronauts, Olympic athletes, and now you. Are you ready?

Affirmations

This is your positive mind, positive vibe essential. You will learn how this simple tool can switch up your life so much. Affirmations follow these three simple rules: They must be positive, personal, and present. As discussed above, it doesn't matter one bit if you don't believe it. You will, and it will become second nature. People sometimes think singing their own praises or saying how great they are is almost viewed as a negative attribute. Guess what? You will come up against enough people in your life who will happily tear you down. You don't need to be one of them. So let's get started. Firstly, let's think of an area you are struggling with. For me, it was my health that was getting me down and just my general negative thinking. So I started there. But it could be relationships, money, self-esteem, or just feeling generally overwhelmed. When you first start, it can be a struggle to think of something. Every day, I used Pinterest for inspiration, listened to affirmations on YouTube, and read Louise Hay's book *You Can Heal Your Life*. You can find links to all of this in the back of the book, including links to my own Pinterest page, where there's loads of inspiring affirmations.

I would google affirmations for health, affirmations for positive thinking, and just general affirmations.

I would pick one for the day and use it. Upon waking, say the affirmation; throughout the day when you feel stressed, overwhelmed, or panicked, say the affirmation. Your head will tell you, *Don't be stupid; what are you talking about,* but do it. Do it. Do it. Push through the negative backchat. You're training your brain after years of being mean to yourself. It will take time, but it will happen. You'll walk past a mirror one day and think, *Hmmm, I look nice,* or *I totally rock.*

I have grouped some affirmations into areas you may be working with. Dip in; pick what works for you. There are so many available online, and come time, you'll create your own.

Affirmations for Health

I love myself, and I am perfectly healthy.

Every day is a new day of hope, happiness, and health.

I am full of energy and vitality, and my mind is calm and peaceful.

I am healthy, healed, and whole.

Every cell in my body vibrates with energy and health.

I take loving care of my body, and my body responds with health.

Affirmations for Relationships (Love, Family, Friends)

I deserve loving relationships and find love with ease.

My marriage is becoming stronger, deeper, and more stable each day.

I am blessed with an incredible family and wonderful friends.

The perfect partner is coming for me sooner than I expect.

I forgive those who have hurt me in the past and move away from them with ease.

People enjoy being with me because I'm a joyful person.

I am so grateful to have supportive [friends, partner, family].

I listen closely and open my heart when interacting with others.

Affirmations for Career/Work

I am creating the career of my dreams.
I deserve a job that fulfils me, and I am now ready to find it.
Today, I see ways this job contributes to my [happiness, wealth, growth].
Today and every day, I use my talents in fulfilling ways.
I am passionate in my career, and it rewards me with monetary freedom.
My work is enjoyable and fulfilling, and I am appreciated.
I make a valued contribution, and my contribution is valued.

Affirmations Money/Wealth

I love money, and it flows easily into my life.
I am debt free, and money is constantly flowing into my life.
Positive thinking attracts money into my life.
Attracting money is easy.
I pay my bills with ease.
I deserve to be wealthy.

Affirmations for Leisure and Creativity

I am creating a harmonious life.
I always make time to relax.
I create harmony in my life by creating a balanced lifestyle.
I fill my leisure time with healthy, enjoyable activities.
I make time to play, relax, and have fun.

Exercise 1: Find an affirmation that works for you. Write it on a Post-it, and put it beside your bed so it will be the first thing you see in the morning. Upon waking, say it. Set it as a reminder on your phone so it will pop up at a certain time daily. You could even save it as a screen saver on your computer. The more you say it, the more your brain will believe it. Repetition is key. Anything can remind you to use your affirmation. Remind yourself how amazing you truly are.

It's the repetition of affirmations that leads
to belief. And once that belief becomes a
deep conviction, things begin to happen.
—Muhammad Ali

Your Cue to Switch

You'll become more aware of the chat you have with yourself. Now is the time to get it to stop. If it's not serving you, benefitting you, or helping you feel better, it has to stop. Here's the deal: Every time one of these sneaky, mean thoughts appears to you, do something to switch the thought process. Do something that will prevent you from getting sucked in and pulled down the negative spiral of the inner critic.

Here's what I did: Every time a little voice would say, "Oh, Susi, you're so obviously going to fail at that," or whatever else rubbish it had decided to throw at me that day, I would say—are you ready for this? This one will make you laugh—I would rap, yip, you heard me: rap. And the song I would rap was Vanilla Ice's "Ice Ice Baby." I'd say in my head a firm "Stop, collaborate, and listen. Ice is back with a brand-new edition." Never ever had to go much further than that, as it was enough to make me laugh and get the stop in there before the negative chat took over. It could be anything, though. Maybe the Spice Girls ("Stop right now; thank you very much") or the Supremes ("Stop in the name of love, before you break my heart"), or I've even had client sing "Jingle Bells." Anything that will halt the negative talk in its tracks. Have you got the idea? Get creative; have fun with it, and see what works for you.

Exercise 2: Create your cue, have fun with it, and laugh. After you create your cue, use it. You'll be surprised at first how many times you find yourself using it. Then as your positive mindset grows, your need for the cue will decrease. So awesome and so simple.

Case Study: Ruth: Ruth is 57, works full-time in a service job, always giving to others; she is in a relationship but has no children. Ruth was searching for a solution to break her negative thought patterns.

Having suffered from an eating disorder in her teens and early adult life, her self-confidence and self-worth were at a huge low. She'd dipped in and out of meditation but never felt like she knew what she was doing. Having experienced bereavements throughout her life, she worried, was feeling anxious, and was overthinking. Time on her own allowed her to sit with her thoughts, which were frequently unhealthy ones.

She came to me, thinking that she'd never have a positive relationship with herself or others, believing she wasn't great at her job, and was regularly experiencing some form of drama in her life. Fast-forward two and a half years from our first meeting.

Ruth has wholeheartedly embraced the ten steps and is living a life she would describe as calm, peaceful, and one where even her family and partner have commented on the positive changes in her.

The first step for Ruth was to embrace the mindset work. To this day, she still uses daily affirmations to influence and support a positive day. She spent years in a relationship that was unhealthy to her physical body, and her mental health had suffered.

Ruth credits her transformation today to recognising her self-worth again, prioritising herself and retraining her brain into letting herself know she was important. She now wants to take care of her beautiful body through eating well and regular yoga classes.

She's created healthy boundaries for herself and manages to detach from the drama of others and step back. Meditation and visualisation supported this mental shift.

Ruth can now look at a positive outcome; she can look at situations objectively and without judgement. She is more aware of spending time in nature and can see the world as a beautiful and inspiring place. She loves, crystals, essential oils, and breath work and has recently trained to be a reiki practitioner. She's done all this in two years. She's created a life free from anxiety, stress, and oppression to one she loves. She has become her own best friend.

Be free, Ruth.

Visualisations

Create the highest, grandest vision possible for your life, because you become what you believe.
—Oprah Winfrey

This mental practice can help you realise your hopes and achieve your dreams and desires, whether that be the ability to get out of bed in the morning, do a presentation at work, or climb Kilimanjaro. Visualisation will allow you to turn your thoughts into a reality. The saying "Be careful what you wish for because you just might get it" is so true.

You may think this idea is new to you. But if you have experienced anxiety, stress, panic, or depression, you're probably a visualisation expert. We visualise and run through all the scenarios of something happening, everything that could go wrong, why we couldn't do something. Have you done this? I used to do this with pretty much every situation. I'd create scenarios in my brain, thinking about all the worst outcomes, what people were thinking, how people would react, completely overplaying a situation that hadn't even occurred yet. This is our brain, trying to protect us, save ourselves from rejection, but actually, it's creating a whole host of negative reactions within our body, both mental and physical. It's time to hone this skill to benefit our lives.

Angie LeVann, resilience coach and speaker, says, "Brain studies now reveal that thoughts produce the same mental instructions as actions. Mental imagery impacts many cognitive processes in the brain: motor control, attention, perception, planning, and memory. So, the brain is getting trained for actual performance during visualisation. It's been found that mental practices can enhance motivation, increase confidence and self-efficacy, improve motor performance, prime your brain for success, and increase states of flow—all relevant to achieving your best life!"

So what does that mean? Well, if we think of something happening, our body responds as if it is. This has been demonstrated in numerous studies where some people visualised going to the gym and others actually went to the gym. Both groups increased their muscle mass. This technique is used by athletes, including Tiger Woods. Famous people such as Oprah Winfrey and Jim Carrey attribute their success to visualisation.

So how do we do it in a positive way? Let's think of a standard day. You wake in the morning, press snooze maybe once, maybe three times, and drag yourself out of bed to face yet another day at work. Does that sound familiar? Maybe you are a morning person already. But let's just tune into how that feels. How does your body feel? Can you imagine it all warm in bed, the dread in your chest about getting up and facing another dull day? OK, let's switch it. Now imagine hearing the alarm going off, and this time stretching and thinking, *Great, another awesome day.* You feel yourself smiling; your chest feels soft and warm and open. Your heart is filled with joy, and your mind feels clear. You imagine everything at work going your way, and you leave work in time to have a beautiful meal with friends.

No dread, no imaging your boss being lousy, no roads being busy.

OK, so that's it in super simple format, and it really can be that easy. Here's how to get visualisation to work in your favour. You can do this for absolutely any situation, big or small, from meeting with friends, picking healthy foods, feeling confident, trying something new, or starting your own business. Visualisation will help you get there and really feel what it's like to live the life you deserve and desire.

The key to visualisation is to really engage your senses:

- What can you see? Look around you in your visualisation; take it all in. Who's with you? Where are you?
- What can you hear? Is there music, nature sounds, people talking or singing?
- What can you smell? Does this situation have a specific smell?
- How do you feel in your body? Where do you feel it in your body? Does your body feel alert or calm, excited or relieved?

Fully engage with it all. I love making a vision board. This allows me to tune in on a daily basis with what motivates me, inspires me, and lifts me up. It's a place where you can add pictures of things related to your visualisation. If your visualisation is to overcome anxiety, you may have pictures of things you'd love to do, calming images, and pictures of people looking healthy, vibrant, confident: things that will make you feel healthy and vibrant. Words and phrases to support this vision or powerful quotes to help keep you focused. This is super fun and really gets you tuning into your desired feelings and desired life.

Exercise 3: Pick a situation or goal that you may have. Picture or visualise it coming to fruition, going exactly as planned. Yes, exactly as planned, no Ifs, ands, or buts, and no catastrophic outcomes. Only good, positive, and supportive outcomes. Run it like a movie in your mind. But it's a spectacular blockbuster, 4-D, with all the senses being engaged. Do this every day for a week and see what evolves from this practice.

I love using visualisation for all sorts of things. It's a great way to allow positive things to happen and life to flow with ease.

Tapping EFT

This was something I had no experience of until my thirties. Tapping via the Emotional Freedom Technique (EFT) calms the nervous system, rewires the brain, and restores balance within the body. As the name suggests, tapping involves tapping on specific areas of the body. These areas that you tap stimulate meridian end points, points used in acupuncture and acupressure. Tapping can really help us overcome emotional blocks or triggers that are holding us back. It helps release them, cleans up our past thoughts, and allows us to live our life fully and in the present moment. Tapping helps reprogramme the amygdala in the brain, which controls our fight-or-flight response. It's a wonderful way to overcome any fears.

When I first discovered tapping, I had some reservations and struggled with it. Here's why: We affirm what is going on. I felt like I was drawing attention to all the things I wanted to forget. I'd worked super hard on being positive, so why would I suddenly start focusing on what was causing me pain, discomfort, or anxiety? Nick Ortner, author of *The Tapping Solution*, asked that very question to the queen of positivity and affirmations, Louise Hay.

Here was her response: "Honey, if you want to clean a house, you got to see the dirt." This showed me clarity and a totally new perspective. Overcoming our fear, anxieties, stress, and depression is not about pretending it's not there; it's about acknowledging, experiencing, and releasing.

So how do we tap? Tapping follows a specific sequence. I started by following some YouTube videos; I did more research and then practised myself. You can now find many loving and supportive practitioners who can assist you with this practice. It's truly fascinating and really empowering when I find myself subconsciously tapping when I'm feeling particularly stressed. There's some links to some tapping resources at the end of this book. You'll also find my tapping tutorial on YouTube.

Tapping Points

Karate chop point on side of hand, top of head, eyebrow near your nose, corner outside of the eye, under eye, under nose, chin, collarbone, under arm, wrist, thumb, each finger, back to karate chop point. This can be easily remembered, as after you tap the karate chop point, the points travel down the body.

We begin by bringing our attention to an area we're struggling with. We need to keep it really specific. It may be something like experiencing anxiety in a public place, rather than your anxiety as a whole. So we identify the issue. Then we close our eyes and really tune in to how this makes us feel, where we feel it in our body, what emotions arise when we think about it: anger, frustration, sadness. We then rate the issue from 1–10 in intensity, 1 being great and 10 affecting you a great deal. Then we begin.

We start by tapping the fleshy part of our hand at the karate chop point. We do this continuously whilst repeating the starting phrase. The starting phrase is "Even though I have this _____, I deeply and completely accept myself."

For example, if using the issue above, it would be "Even though I have this anxiety in public places, I deeply and completely accept myself." Repeat it three times.

Then we move onto the reminder phrase, which is maybe something along the lines of "This anxiety of public places has been blocking me," or "I feel this anxiety is harming me," and we would tap our way through the points, tapping between three and seven times on each point. So for the pain example, you could use "This pain," "This pain has been holding me back," "This pain is overwhelming me," "Even though I have this pain, I deeply and completely accept myself."

As you go through the sequence, some emotions or thoughts related to the experience may arise. Allow them to surface and acknowledge them.

After this sequence, we would use more positive phrases. "This anxiety is making me stronger," "I know there is a lesson in this emotional experience," "I am not my anxiety," "My anxiety does not control me," "I choose to release this anxiety."

Once you have completed the sequence, stop, take a deep breath in, and then slowly exhale. Tune into yourself again, and now rate the issue again. Has your score changed? If it has decreased, wonderful. You can continue to use this technique until your discomfort is reduced.

- Identify the issue.
- Rate the issue.
- Follow the tapping sequence and wording.
- Review and rate the issue again.

Exercise 4: Select the main issue you would like help with. Head over to my YouTube channel, and follow along with me, doing the tapping as described above. If you don't have access to a computer, no problem at all. Follow the simple steps above in order, replacing the phrases to align with your issue. Want to know more about these techniques? See the recommended reading at the back of this book.

Your mind is ready. These techniques will serve you forever, not just in times of difficulty. They will become habits and tools that you reach for every day in life, assisting you to see the truth, beauty, and all that you deserve.

Repeat, repeat, repeat.

NOTES PAGE

Chapter 2
The Good, the Bad, and the Ugly: Protecting Yourself from Negativity

I surround myself with joy and optimism, I allow only that which is good and positive to enter my being.

When we are already in a negative mindset, or one where negativity can take control, protecting ourselves from any external negativity is an essential coping mechanism to learn. This chapter allows us to identify areas where we can pick up on energies which aren't our own; it shows how these can affect us and how to protect ourselves from them. Following these principles allows us to live a more positive life, making choices to support our own happiness.

A negative mind brings a negative life. A positive mind brings a positive life. What we feed our minds is so important. In 2014, as I lay in bed, ill, I found that watching the news would upset me, listening to friends complain about boyfriends and parking tickets would leave me feeling wiped, reading celebrity magazines about divorce, affairs, and the red carpet left me sad.

What I discovered was that I already had enough negativity going on in my own mind. I didn't need to take on anybody else's.

When we are in an anxious, stressed, or depressed state, we are really vulnerable to picking up on the negativity and emotions of others. This may be a concept you've explored before. I'm sure you've had the experience of being around a certain person, and when you leave them, you feel drained and your mood has shifted. One of my clients, Wendy, calls these people mood hoovers. I'm sure you have one of those in your life. Or have you been in a lousy mood but then you spend time catching up with a friend who is uplifting and inspiring, and you feel instantly better, and your spirits lifted. The latter is the person you need to be around just now.

When we feel the emotions of others, this is called empathy. Being empathetic can be a blessing and a curse. It's beautiful that we can really feel how others are feeling and know what they are going through. This makes us a wonderful supporter who can truly understand others. It allows us to really be there for friends and family. The downside to this is you may be worry about someone's issue, long after it has crossed their mind. They may have moved on and continued with their lives, yet you are left with the energy associated to this.

This super sensitivity to others can really affect us mentally, emotionally, and even physically.

Are You an Empath?

- Do you feel you can be in tune with others and connect with what they are thinking?
- When a friend or family member is in pain, do you sometimes feel it too?
- Do you cry when you see sad things on TV?
- Do you find it easy to talk about your moods and emotions?
- Do you struggle with confrontation?
- Do complete strangers find it easy to talk to you and confide in you?
- Do you feel physically sick when you hear something upsetting on the news?
- Do you feel drawn to nature and animals?

If you answered yes to these questions, then there is every likelihood that you are an empath. Being an empath is such a beautiful gift in life, but we do need to manage and support this trait, or else it can become overbearing.

A lot of my clients are empaths, suffering from trying to do too much for other people, help others, support others, and save everyone else from suffering whilst taking it all on themselves. Can you relate? I think most of us who suffer from anxiety, agitation, and low mood take the world on our shoulders and lack support ourselves. We lack the ability to make ourselves a priority. This is why it's so important to learn how to separate our own suffering from that of others.

Protecting your mind, body, and soul from the energy of others is so important. As a healer, I regularly feel what others are going through; sometimes, I have a day where I'm feeling a bit off, and I don't know why; I realise that I'm actually feeling somebody else's emotions. Protecting ourselves is so important. I've learnt this the hard way. I often have clients who come to me, and when we do their treatment and clear their energy, it was heavy around them; we realise that this heaviness wasn't theirs to be carrying. I have a number of rituals and routines I use to support protecting my energy and also clearing the energy of others.

For some, this may seem a bit woo-woo and crazy, but others may already be aware of it. But in simple terms, have you ever gone into work or been around family, and when you've gone in, you felt great, excited, and happy, but by the time you leave, you feel drained and exhausted? Not because you've been upset or sad about something, but just being in that environment has affected you. These simple tools and tricks will help protect you and clear your energy.

Bubble of Light

This is a super simple and lovely way of protecting your energy. I use this every morning. You can do this in bed before you even get out of bed and open your eyes. You visualise yourself surrounded in a beautiful golden or white bubble. This bubble protects you from all forms of negativity; they can't get near you or enter your being. Nasty comments and other emotions will simply be reflected away like a mirror or bounce off. This is a wonderful tool for all ages. This is a great one to use if you know you are about to enter a potentially negative situation or be around a negative person. Applying this prior to entering or being around that person will assist you in protecting yourself from negativity.

Detox Bath

Bathing in Epsom or Himalayan salts is a wonderful way of clearing any negative energy around you. Water and salt are both wonderful energy clearers and cleansers. By simply lying and relaxing in a bath, you can help your energy feel super sparkly and awesome. For your detox bath, run a warm bath and add around 200 grams or more of salts (adding a couple drops of essential oils to your salts can make it extra relaxing). Bathe for twenty minutes before washing your hair or adding any extra products. Then once you're finished, shower your body to rinse all the salts away. Great for energy clearing and has so many other additional benefits too (see "Flying Solo," Chapter 9, for more on this magical method of bathing).

Shower of Positivity

If you don't have time or cannot bathe, this is a great option for clearing negativity. You can do this as a visualisation as well as a real-life action. This is a great end-of-day activity or coming home from work, if your work has left you feeling stressed or overwhelmed. As you stand in the shower, water falling over you, you first start to imagine that the water is washing all your cares and worries down the drain. With every drop of water, you feel your worries disappear. You now begin to imagine that the water is clearing any negativity from your being. The water cleanses you and clears you and leaves you feeling more like you, back to a neutral feeling. I then like to imagine the shower changing, and it showers you in beautiful droplets of positivity. I like to visualise these as golden, but it can be any colour that resonates with you. You finish your shower feeling clearer, more positive, and relaxed.

Sage or Frankincense Oil Smudging

I regularly cleanse my home and body from negativity using these fabulous natural cleansers. Both of these have been used as a method of spiritual cleansing and clearing for thousands of years. I love using both, and switch between the two, although frankincense has a less offensive smell and is smoke free.

White Sage

The first time I purchased this, I bought some online after reading it was great for clearing negativity. As my head was in such a dark place, I thought I'd try anything. I hid in my bathroom and lit this magical bundle of what looks like dried herbs. The smell really shocked me. It reminded me of being a student or being at parties when I was younger, and people would be getting stoned in a corner. A little bit panicky, I opened my bathroom window, allowing the fragrant smell of sage to float out into the street. My husband could smell this weird smell and was a little alarmed at what I was up to next, on my path to being anxiety free. I remember this night so well; it actually brings tears to my eyes, laughing. So be prepared if you haven't yet met with the wonders of sage. I now use this in my home if there has been any illness or arguments to shift the energy, and it's also antibacterial. Double-win.

To use the sage, you get a bundle, light the end, and allow it to smoulder. Hold your sage bundle over a plate or shell (this is the traditional vessel) to prevent any falling off and burning your carpet or floor. Once you have the sage smouldering, you can waft the smoke around your body, under your arms and feet and the outside area of your body, cleansing and clearing away any negative energy.

Frankincense

Frankincense wasn't an essential oil I was familiar with until my mum was diagnosed with cancer. I'd heard of it from the Bible's Christmas story, but that was about it. Frankincense is a hugely powerful and beneficial essential oil that's regarded by many as the king of oils, due to its many uses and benefits. I had researched this oil a lot during my mum's cancer journey; during this research, I discovered that this oil was particularly great for spiritually and energetically cleansing and purifying areas. Frankincense is also a wonderful tool for helping reduce anxiety and elevate the mood. I love to use this ritual at bedtime to clear any energy that's lingering and then help ease me into a restful sleep. The properties in frankincense keep us calm, grounded, and connected.

To perform this cleansing ritual, I apply a drop of frankincense oil to my palms. I rub them together and take a deep inhale. Then starting from my head, I gently wave my hands around my body. Moving from head, front, and back of body, along the lengths of my arms and under my arms, legs, and soles of feet. You can see a how-to video for this on my YouTube channel. I then stroke the palms of my hands across the back of my neck to finish. You can also diffuse frankincense if you feel the energy is off in your home, but this is my go-to clearing option for me.

Exercise 1: Protect your energy each morning using the Bubble of Light tool above; pick one of the energy clearing rituals above, and use it three times this week. Or mix and match to find out what suits you best. Starting from a neutral point is always best; it's even better if we can also increase our feelings of positivity.

Psychology

Pour in the positivity; keep it coming and flowing. Another reason we need to fill ourselves up with so much positivity is, as humans, we are affected by cognitive bias. Cognitive bias is where our brains jump to a conclusion or answer. This protective measure is a way for our brains to reduce our decision making. However, if we have already got stuck in a negative thinking pattern, this will be our brain's immediate go-to response. For example, you're walking down a dark street and see some shadows across the street. You immediately think it's a person or attacker, rather than logically reasoning that it's just the shadow of the wheelie bin. You see two people whispering, and assume it's obviously about you.

Whilst at Ohio State University, Dr John Cacioppo discovered another human cognitive bias, known as "negativity bias." Without becoming a science geek, simply put, this means your brain is more sensitive to negative information than positive, whether that be through pictures, words, or actions. What was further demonstrated by this bias is that you need to experience more positive experiences than negative. So unfortunately, it's not balanced. In fact, it is suggested that you need five positive experiences or interactions to one negative.

This explains why it's sometimes so hard to shake off something someone has said to you. Have you ever gotten feedback about something, and all you can think of is the one bad thing they said? Your partner makes a nice dinner and surprises you, but all you can focus on is the mess in the kitchen. You had an argument years ago, and you still can't shake off the feelings. These are all examples of negativity bias.

So wonderful psychology is stacked against us from the outset. What can we do to prevent ourselves from continuously being drawn down this negative route? The answer is creating more positive experiences and thoughts than negative. We have to rewire our brains to create positive neural pathways. Sound complicated? It's easier than you think.

Gratitude

We can begin to rewire the brain simply by weaving in more positive experiences. One of my favourite ways to do this is creating a gratitude practice. I recommend it to all my clients.

We often move through our everyday lives without truly paying attention to the beauty and positive experiences around us. Life gets busy and overwhelming. We're racing from one thing to the next, with little consideration for what wondrous things have happened in the here and now.

When life is tough, we sometimes feel that there has been no joy; no good things happen. It's easy to get caught in the downwards spiral of negativity and sadness. I first started my daily gratitude practice when I was bedridden; seriously, to begin with, it was so hard. I was in such a dark place, and it was a real struggle to focus on joy. I can't even remember where I got the idea, but I started a gratitude jar. Every day, I would write something I was grateful for on a piece of paper and then pop that paper into my jar. I've shared some of my little notes below:

January 10. Saw beautiful rainbows brighter than I've ever seen.

January 11. Had the most wonderful bath.

January 12. Cuddling Lili and watching a *Barbie* movie.

January 20. Got my power and confidence going on. I love life.

Start with the little things we are grateful for; it

can seem pretty insignificant, even having a nice cup of tea. But the acknowledgment of all the small things is key. The small things are often all we have when times are tough. In Rick Hanson's Ted Talk, "Hardwiring Happiness," he explains we need to stay with the good experiences for longer. We can change our brain and inner strength simply by recognising and staying with the good experiences for longer. The key time to spend is ten to twenty seconds recognising the good thing in order for it to affect our brains.

This is why I suggest writing down the things you are grateful for, as opposed to just making a mental note. You can get lots of wonderful pretty journals you can use. Or as I started, you can simply grab some scrap paper and an old jar and begin there. Start small, with recognising one thing a day, then work your way up to three a day. This is sometimes easier than others. Every day may not be good, but there will be something good in every day. I gifted my mum a gratitude jar I had made when she was going through her cancer journey. It's a wonderful thing visually, as you can begin to see all the good things growing. It's a nice thing to reach for when you're having a difficult day to reread some of what you have written.

Every day may not be good, but there will be something good in every day.

35

Gratitude is going to be one of the most powerful tools you have. When anxious, depressed, or stressed, it can feel like there is no light at the end of the tunnel; however, focusing on what we have as opposed to what we don't is one of the many keys to happiness. I still do this as a daily practice and find it keeps me mindful and focused on the joy around me.

Dr David Hamilton, author of the book *The Five Effects of Kindness*, claimed the following ten benefits from starting and maintaining a gratitude practice:

1. It's good for mental health. People who have a regular gratitude practice are 25 per cent happier than those who don't.
2. It helps counter stress. Gratitude helps take your mind away from stress and frustration. It helps you notice more of the good things.
3. It inspires you to exercise more. A 2003 study of people who kept a weekly gratitude practice found they exercised more.
4. It helps you achieve your goals. Research over a two-month period showed that people making gratitude lists were found to be more likely to make progress towards important personal goals.

5. It makes you kinder. One finding of gratitude research is that people keeping daily gratitude lists are more likely to help someone in need.

6. It makes you feel less lonely and more connected. Being more kind also improves your relationships and connections with others. Some participants in gratitude studies indeed report feeling more connected to people. Some people practicing gratitude also feel more connected and part of life as a whole. It increases their sense of belonging in the world.

7. It helps you sleep better. I recommend doing your gratitude practice before heading to bed. Moving your mind to a positive place before sleep and focusing on the good helps you to relax, making falling to sleep much easier.

8. It makes you feel more in control of your life. Gratitude has a positive effect on your whole life, renewing optimism and allowing you to feel more in control of your emotions and the situations life throws at you.

9. People like you better. Bringing awareness to the people you love and are grateful for can transform your relationships. It allows you to see the best in yourself and others. It can make you more considerate to others. This can often be

enough for people to be feel more valued and enjoy your relationships more.

10. It leads to better health. Some studies have even shown that gratitude boosts your overall physical and cardiovascular health. It boosts your immune system and can even lower blood pressure.

Exercise 2: Start a gratitude practice of your own. It can be super simple, by keeping a notebook and pen by your bedside table. Or you could create a gratitude jar using my free printable Gratitude Jar Making project (www.spiritandsoul.me). Making a jar can be really fun and is a great thing to do with children too. It's a really simple craft idea that won't take long and can really change your life and boost your mood. Either way, make a start, and watch how your joy shifts.

Gratitude is a daily practice that opens your eyes to the joy around you. It really transforms your day when you are more mindful, grateful, and happy to be alive.

Case Study: Nicola. Nicola came to see me when she was 22. Her father had seen an article about my story in the local press and thought I may be able to help. Nicola was teacher training at the time and spending her life travelling between two cities. She had a busy life: university, family, boyfriend, but she had become overwhelmed by it all.

Having previously suffered from an eating disorder, Nicola was fully aware how easy it was for her life to spiral out of control. Her need to control the chaos found some comfort from food and then exercise to excess, to balance the eating.

It had reached crisis point after a negative experience during an overseas placement. Her anxiety was now through the roof, and panic was common. Nicola had lost all confidence in herself and her ability to cope. She had reached a point where her thinking was so negative that harming herself seemed like the only solution. Thankfully, Nicola sought professional help from her GP and started medication to support her treatment.

This option worked and allowed her to reach a plateau of managing her conditions, but she felt it was like sticking a plaster on an even larger problem. She was seeking long-term solutions, and that's where our journey began.

Her first visit to see me, Nicola had got her boyfriend to drive the night before with her, making sure she knew where she was going and to alleviate the fear of something new. She initially came to see me for meditation classes, and she still does, to this day. The transformation from that first fearful day to today is profound.

Nicola had never meditated in her life prior to meeting me; now this is one of her go-to tools for remaining calm, staying in control, and keeping things in perspective.

Before attending classes, her brain was focused on highlighting anything that wasn't going right; from sleeping in to being stuck in traffic, it would be enough to completely overwhelm her and throw her off. Now Nicola has the ability to take a step back, to see the big picture, and she has a greater perspective of life and what's important to her.

The key area that has supported Nicola the most has been becoming aware of negative energy. Before, she would get sucked into the cycle of negative thinking, looking for others to validate her. She enjoyed others agreeing just how bad things were. From attending classes, she realised that she needed to take a step back from those who fed her doom-and-gloom cycle. As she embraced more positive thinking in her life, things began to change and improve. Some people didn't like this new positive person, but Nicola discovered it was not her job to change the thinking of others. It was her job to change her own outlook.

What was Nicola's number one tool to overcome

negativity? Gratitude. Gratitude allowed her to find contentment where she was in her life. It allowed her to fall in love with her body and exercise again, leading from her heart and nourishing her body. If overwhelming feelings kick in, Nicola looks at the things she's grateful for: her education, her family, and her love of being in nature. She had forgotten how much joy the little things in life brought her. Now, if something doesn't go to plan, Nicola uses mindfulness and gratitude to allow her to see the bigger picture.

Nicola has rediscovered her confidence, value in herself, and love of life. She's amazing.

Be free, Nicola.

Mood Hoovers and Negative Nellies

I'm sure you've had that one friend or colleague in your lifetime who when you're around them, you instantly feel drained. Yep, you know who I'm talking about. This person can even be a family member or even your spouse. The more aware you become of how you feel and how negative your life has gotten, the more you see the negativity that surrounds you. As hard as it is, when you are trying to overcome your own anxiety and low mood, you really do need to protect yourself from the moods of others.

This doesn't even have to be personal contact. We often get depleted by things such as the news, a Facebook feed, or even an email. What is depleting you? Once we know, we can begin to do something about it. It's not a case of banishing them from your life; this isn't always possible. It's about increasing your positive interactions and reducing your negative ones.

When my mum was going through her cancer journey, she loved social media as a way to connect with friends and family from her bed. However, she found that one person's feed really upset her. This person was so negative online that it left Mum feeling upset. So I encouraged her to unfollow that person.

If an online presence or story upsets you, there are many options to take. You can organise your Facebook feed to show information from positive pages and groups so the first things you see are uplifting. You can unfollow people who are draining you or don't make you feel good. This doesn't mean unfriend, as I said earlier; it's tricky if it's a family member. But by unfollowing, you will only see something if you directly go and look. Having a social media clear-up is always a good idea.

In-person interactions can be trickier. You may find this person looks to you for support, that they are unwilling to take responsibility for what's going on for them in their own lives. They may be the victim in their lives, always a drama, always a story. They are almost seeking your love and assurance but fail to see what you are going through yourself. Can you think of anyone? This person may be super opinionated or judgemental of others, and you find their constant judgement really draining or negative. Or the final one, one I recently had to step back from, is someone who makes you feel disempowered, who is competitive with you, or you just have a feeling they don't make you feel good. You don't need to have a reason or even an exact experience, but someone not making you feel good is enough to stop interacting with them.

The key is to keep situations light and limit the interactions if you can. Step back and spend less time with these types. If possible, you can stop contact altogether. This is time for you to put your own needs first, to build yourself up and increase your positive experiences. If you do need to still interact with your negative Nellies, then you can agree to meet in a neutral place; set a time and explain you have something else on after, so you are in control of how much time you spend with them.

I'm not saying only surround yourself with positive people, but what I am saying is, be careful. We all go through difficult times: death, loss, illness, relationship issues, and it's important to support ourselves and friends through these times. But it's those who actually have a pretty good life and continue to moan and take from you, that you need to restrict.

Do you have supporters in your group or circle? Do you have people who leave you feeling inspired and held? These can be friends, relatives, colleagues, or even people you follow online or social media, who fill your cup with positivity. For me, my sister, my mum when she was alive, my best friend Erika Cowie, and all my clients inspire me and allow me to feel supported. Online, I love to follow Louise Hay, Oprah, Rachel Hollis, and other empowering women to raise my spirits and keep my mood high. This leads to a constant exchange in energy. There needs to be balance. I personally listen to podcasts or read something inspiring every day of my life. I constantly fill my bucket with positivity. This is the key.

Exercise 3: This exercise is about awareness. Spend some thinking about who or what it is that lifts you up and who or what it is that leaves you feeling drained. Once you have this awareness, you can look to build on the positive and reduce the negative exposure. Starting with social media is a great way to begin to get you thinking and making changes. This exercise is about putting your needs first. Find your energy and reclaim it back.

Volunteering

I regularly volunteer my time. I used to work with a charity once a month, spending time with a young boy who was struggling due to his family life. I have helped with Riding for the Disabled, assisting in helping children with physical and mental disabilities ride ponies. As a family, we do an annual beach clear-up, where we clear our local beach and then have a BBQ at our home. And lastly, I currently offer my time for free in my local area taking mindful beach walks. These walks are donation based, and the money goes to our local charity to help allow beach access for people with wheelchairs and helps finance local events throughout the year.

All these activities require is time. So often, we race through life, thinking we don't have time to support anyone else; this often isn't the case. We should value the act of giving. It can be any amount of time. Even donating blood is an act of supporting and giving for the greater good.

Volunteering not only makes a difference to those you are helping; it can also have a positive impact on your own physical and mental health.

From my own personal experience, volunteering allowed me to connect with others, develop my social interactions, and push me that little bit outside my comfort zone, but with the knowledge that my help and support was needed. It allowed me to develop my confidence after I had lost it. It allowed me to add more value to my own life. It got me out of a place where I felt my life was awful to feeling more grateful.

Studies have shown that volunteering can lower levels of anxiety, decrease depression, and reduce stress. Volunteering has been shown to decrease your risk of dementia and heart disease. It reduces feelings of social isolation and loneliness. Volunteering has even been shown to reduce levels of chronic pain and illness. What's even more incredible is, research suggest that those who volunteer actually gain more health benefits than those who are receiving the help.

The Corporation for National and Community Service in America reports, "Volunteer activities can strengthen the social ties that protect individuals from isolation during difficult times, while the experience of helping others leads to a sense of greater self-worth and trust."

With so much to gain and the knowledge that you will be making a difference to lives of others, what should you do? Lots of charities rely on the support of volunteers. What interests do you have? Mental health awareness, animals, and the environment can all benefit from your volunteering efforts. Maybe you have a family history of a condition and want to give back to help others in a similar situation. There are so many sponsored events which can offer goals and purpose. There's an option for everyone.

Exercise 4: Think about what your interests are and research locally, nationally, or internationally and see what you could do to help. Maybe it's an hour a week or even an hour a year. Your help is valued. See how you feel. It really is a huge win-win situation.

Random Acts of Kindness

Little gestures can make a huge difference, from a stranger holding a door to a friend giving you a compliment to a neighbour scraping your driveway in the snow. These simple and free acts of kindness can make a huge difference to another person's day.

You never fully know what another person is going through. If I saw someone really grumpy or snappy, I would think they were just downright rude. It wasn't really until Mum was given her terminal cancer diagnosis that I was fully aware of how hard it can be to be out in public whilst your world is falling apart. My sister and I actually had this conversation; it was a huge realisation to us both.

That mum screaming at her kids in the supermarket could have just lost her husband; that driver who is speeding could be on the way to a hospital; that person moaning about the prices in front of you could have just been fired. We truly never know how life is for someone else.

What I do know is that when we do small acts of kindness, it not only makes the other person feel great; it can also reduce negative aspects of our own lives.

While I wrote this book, my 9-year-old decided to use her own money to make up bags to give the homeless at Christmas. In these bags Lili put snacks, water, toiletries, fruit, sweets and gloves and hats to keep them warm on the streets. This brought her such happiness, and as she handed them out, she could see the joy that her random act of kindness brought to another human being.

Kindness has been shown to reduce anxiety, pain, stress, and depression whilst increasing joy, happiness, energy, and lifespan. The beauty of kindness is, it's contagious. So sprinkle it around and share it.

Exercise 5: What random acts of kindness can you do? Maybe leave a Post-it with a nice message on it, compliment a stranger, help a friend or neighbour, message a relative to say how much you love them. Try it and see how the world around you changes.

In this chapter, you have seen how much you consume in the form of negative and positive energy; it can have a huge impact on your life. From reducing negative media coverage to writing down all you're grateful for, each of these steps can have an amazing effect on your outlook and mental health. So keep filling yourself up with positive vibes and detoxing the negative. You deserve to feel positive, alive, and joyous.

Notes page

Chapter 3
So What: Saying No and Creating Boundaries

I set loving and healthy boundaries with myself and others; I live a life that honours my values and truth.

Saying no can be so challenging, resulting in setting ourselves unrealistic schedules and placing enormous pressure on ourselves to always be doing the right thing and giving 100 per cent to everything. Guess what? This is not sustainable or achievable. The only thing you will achieve is burnout. So let's dive in and learn how to be enough, be happy, and make decisions that support our own health.

I'll admit it: I went through life being a people pleaser. Hands up if this is you too. I totally get it. I like other people being happy. I can't stand conflict and hate letting people down. But what does this cost you? Your own happiness? Time? Sanity? Health? At work, things would get passed to me because I was always willing to work things out. The kids would ask if they could try new activities, and I'd say yes despite our already busy schedules. I didn't want to disappoint them. I thought, *It's OK; you can find a way.* I'd say yes to going to events I wasn't really interested in. I'd go to movies I didn't want to see. All these little things may seem insignificant, but when you are constantly saying yes to others, you frequently say no to yourself. As you read through this chapter, I'd like to become more aware of all the activities, things, and people you say yes to when you really want to say no.

The more we say yes to others, the more they expect that yes; the value of what we're saying yes to decreases and becomes the norm. Being at work is a perfect example of this. Over time, what may start out as you helping coworkers out when they feel pushed somehow becomes your responsibility. Then you don't realise until further down the line, "Hey, that's not even my job."

> Daring to set boundaries is about having
> the courage to love ourselves even when
> we risk disappointing others.
> —Brene Brown

Being totally honest, this is the area I have found

the most uncomfortable. It is an ingrained behaviour that I still work through. I have to check in with myself regularly. I hate letting people down. Eventually, this constant yessing landed me in bed, unable to walk properly; I was a stressed and anxious mess.

Do you realise that you're doing it? If you're reading this book and feel stressed or anxious, you probably agree to many things, that aren't even yours to say yes to: activities you would never normally think of doing.

Do you want to know a secret? You have a choice. Crazy, isn't it? Did you know you're actually allowed to say no?

We're going to work through this, and if you start putting your own needs first (notice how I say "needs"; not even wants at this point, but needs first), you will feel significantly better.

Stumbling Block to Success Number 1: "Should"

Should. Oh my, how this word has controlled my life and thoughts throughout the years. Susi, you really should stay up until 1 a.m. and get that piece of work finished. Susi, you really should go into work on a Saturday, or else you'll be behind come Monday. Susi, you really should cook the kids healthier foods. Susi, you really should help in the school library. Susi, you really should go to the gym. Susi, you really should go to Mary's birthday (even though you've only met her twice, are absolutely shattered, and have a ton of other stuff to be doing). Stretch, stretch, stretch. You begin to pull at your energy, at your spirit, and you get lost in a sea of yessing to the expectations others have of you.

In Louise Hay's book *You Can Heal Your Life*, Louise says, "I believe should is one of the most damaging words in our language. Every time we use the word *should*, we are in effect, saying 'wrong.' Either we are wrong, or we were wrong, or we are going to be wrong. I don't think we need any more wrongs in our life."

Our words have so much power, and this little word is a biggie. Take the first example above: "Susi, you should really stay up until 1 a.m. and get that piece of work finished." This is definitely me, saying no to my needs. I'm compromising on my sleep, which then will lead to me being undoubtedly grumpy. I'll probably eat some junk to keep my attention going, even though 1 a.m. is not the best time to have full attention. Doing this piece of work will then lead to an expectation that working at 1 a.m. is perfectly OK or that I can manage my current workload; let's give her some more. Bam, you're caught in a cycle of meeting someone else's (or sometimes even your own) high expectations of yourself.

I put enormous pressure on myself to do and be everything everyone, myself and society, expected of me. Where does this get you? Pleasing everyone, frustrated, and getting further and further away from who you are and what you enjoy.

So what can we do with the dreaded *should* word? We can change it for *could*. This simple switch allows us to have options; it takes our power back and allows us to decide based on our own needs and desires.

Let's look at one of the other examples: "Susi, you really should go to Mary's party." I'd already mentioned above that I barely knew her. What if we change that *should* for *could*? "Susi, you could go to Mary's party". How does that sound? It's such a simple switch, and it releases so much pressure. As people-pleasers, we put an enormous burden on ourselves. Once we switch the *should* for *could*, the next step is making the decision. In this example, will you really be disappointing Mary? Or is this an imagined story you've concocted in your head? As hard as it is, she may have only invited you because of her own people-pleasing tendencies. If you're feeling exhausted, you need to honour that and take a night off, not keep pushing to attend something with someone you barely know. If she's a friend and values you at all, she'll get it.

Exercise 1: For the next week, tune into that internal dialogue again. Become aware of when you use the word *should'* Every time you hear yourself saying the word, switch it up and change it to *could*. See how it feels. Feel into the change. Notice the difference you feel; feel the pressure subside a bit. Acknowledge how much pressure you may have been putting on yourself. This week's exercise is purely to observe and switch. See the freedom and flexibility that this simple switch offers you. Once you recognise your self-criticising ways, you can change them to a more loving and supportive solution.

Case Study: Angela. I met Angela when she approached me for some online meditation work. Based overseas, Angela was early thirties and working in a super stressful job.

She felt she had lost her voice and connection to her soul purpose. In her bid to make everyone else happy, she had forgotten her own happiness.

Angela was blessed that her mum was a complementary therapist and played a huge positive role in supporting her. Having been prescribed antidepressants and antianxiety medication in her late teens, Angela was keen to look at and delve back into the healing and natural options her mum had taught her growing up, to move past the symptoms and look at addressing the root cause. Angela was looking to make lasting, supportive changes.

Angela embraced the full ten steps, becoming aware of nutrition, grounding techniques, meditation, and daily self-care rituals. She maintains regular complementary therapy sessions and has gone on to study further in these areas and become a practitioner in many. She loves Bowen therapy, EFT tapping, reiki, and angel healing, and she's a huge lover and advocate of essential oils.

She has transformed from a loather of movement and exercise to loving running and qualifying as a yin yoga teacher. What an epic and amazing journey she has taken.

How has she managed this? She has learnt to say no and stand up for her beliefs. She created loving boundaries that support her own well-being and growth. This hasn't been easy and has taken practice, focus, and commitment. She makes herself a priority daily. She tunes in to how she feels in situations and honours her inner guidance. By choosing to make her health a priority, she has transformed her life from one of crippling anxiety to one beyond her wildest dreams. She's free from limitations.

Angela now would describe her life as awesome

and empowering. Her confidence and self-worth have grown beyond imagination. She feels she is living a life on purpose, surrounded by those who love and support her. She's truly inspiring and amazing.

Be free, Angela.

So What?

I still use this next part frequently. It's super simple and makes me laugh in a bit of a childish way. I can almost hear my teenage self coming out when I use this tool. You are now growing your awareness of your language and the effect it can have on you. The next stage is looking at the consequence of you saying no. This isn't a deep and highly educated response, but it works get to the core of your inability to say no. When you are beating yourself up re obligations, say, "So what?" It's hilarious but works. Use that teenage tone in your mind. Allow humour to prevail and guide you through your responses. The essence of this exercise is to delve and chat back to your inner critic and self-depreciating talk. Take the pressure off. Time to say, "So what?"

Internal Chat Goes … You Say: "So What"

You took the kids to McDonald's again; you're such a bad parent. You say, "So what?"

You haven't finished that work assignment; you'll be letting your boss down. You say, "So what?"

You didn't go to the movies and see a film (you didn't even like) with a friend. You say, "So what?"

You didn't answer your friend's call, as you knew she would be moaning. You say, "So what?"

You didn't sort out a colleague's mistake for them. "So what?"

Exercise 2: Try this for size. So often when we say yes to things, it's because we worry about the effect of saying no and upsetting people, or not doing as we should. However, in many cases, the consequences are manufactured, do not really exist, or are not as bad as we imagine them to be. Oh, the imagination of an anxiety sufferer. We have the best imaginations, coming up with all sorts of scenarios that may never even occur. Next time you feel an uncomfortable yes coming, "Say no," and ask yourself the question, "So what?" If you give yourself another reason to say yes, then say, "So what?" and another and another and another.

So What, So What, So What, So What, So What, So What, So What?

Here's an example: "Hi, Susi. I wondered if you'd like to come to a party I'm having Friday night."

Susi's thought process: *I should really go; it was nice of her to ask me.* "So what?" *But then she'll think I don't like her.* "So what?" *Other people might notice I'm not there and speak about me.* "So what?" *But I don't want people to speak about me, as it makes me feel uncomfortable.* "So what?"

You get the idea; this could go on and on, reasoning with yourself, but ultimately, it leads you to the real reason you don't want to be there. In this example, it's my fear of being spoken about and not liked. The "people pleaser," not the self-pleaser.

What if we put our own disappointments before the disappointments of others? What if we realise that our time and health are important? Without our health, both mental and physical, we cannot meet any obligations. Depending where you are on your anxiety journey, you may need to be super selfish for a while. This means you come first. When I was really at my lowest, I would still try and push myself to do or go to places that would put my anxiety through the roof. This is so counter-intuitive and will set you back enormously. In order to be free from anxiety, you need to learn to say no.

How to Say No

This is something you need to teach yourself. It may be a word you associate with letting people down or not doing enough. I assure you, once you've learnt how to prioritise your own life and engage back to your own desires, you will find this easier. You will see and feel the benefits. You'll begin to have time for the things and people you love. I had a life coach once say to me, "If it's not a hell yeah, it's a no." So hold that thought as your people-pleasing ways try to pull you further away from your own needs.

First of all, you have nothing to feel guilty for. I'm not saying you won't still feel guilty; you most probably will. But that guilt of saying no will reduce. It's retraining our brain. It's a journey of finding out what we actually like and don't like again, what makes us feel good and what makes us feel uncomfortable.

Your health is hugely important. Your health needs to come first. When your body is telling you no, you need to voice that no for it. When your mind is screaming at you to slow down and rest, you need to voice it. When we override this inner guidance, it becomes outer guidance.

This is when physical and mental ailments appear. I say this from experience: vertigo, panic attacks, back pain, labyrinthitis, chronic conditions, coughs, colds, and even psoriasis over my whole body. Yet I didn't say no until I was left with no option because I was bedridden. My body and mind had had enough and decided to stop working for me and with me.

Learning to say no will be one of the greatest gifts you give yourself.

1. Learning the pause: This will be your first tool to turn to. You may have been automatically saying yes for so long: filling your diary with engagements, over committing, exhausting yourself and stressing out. It will take a little time to retrain your response. Start with the pause. This will allow you to look at your response authentically from your own viewpoint. This gives you time to evaluate if you are saying yes out of obligation or because it is something you genuinely feel will support you. Ways you could incorporate the pause are saying, "Let me double check those dates, and I'll get back to you," and waiting before responding to emails, voicemails, texts, and messages.

2. During the pause, here are some questions you can ask yourself:

   a. Do I really want to do this?

   b. How does saying yes make me feel? Really tune into how doing this activity or piece of work would make you feel. Do you feel happy, stressed, overwhelmed, excited, sick, or tense? Really tune into your internal guidance, your body, and your thoughts.

   c. What will I gain by saying yes? What positive outcome will come from the yes?

   d. If I say no, what will I do with the time?

   e. If I say yes, is it pulling me closer to or further from my goals?

   f. If I say yes, will I feel healthier and more supported or more stressed and overwhelmed?

How to Say No Effectively

No doesn't have to be confrontational or difficult. The reaction we believe others may have to our no is often a fabricated story that we've created from fear. It's always tricky starting something new, and saying no is no exception. Think of saying no as an act of love. To start with, this may seem an unusual concept, but bear with me. Saying no can be an act of self-love, honouring yourself and your needs. It also allows others to get to know and love you better, getting to know the real you. Your ability to be honest with friends, family, and colleagues will develop into greater respect and understanding for you.

Our human nature dictates that we want to be liked and considered kind and caring. But is saying yes when you actually mean no supporting that?

Like any exercise, the more we use it, the easier it becomes. The word loses its power and no longer becomes a scary response. No is a complete answer. You don't need to apologise or explain: "No, I'm not sure," "Maybe next time," or "I would if I could." If you mean no, say no. Are you feeling edgy even reading this? I promise it will get easier. It can be difficult and make you feel uncomfortable. But this short-term feeling of being uncomfortable is so much better than compromising your own needs, desires, and feelings.

Exercise 3: Start saying no. Start by the most basic things, so you can get used to it. Would you like ice in your drink? No. Would you like to come out tonight? No. If you feel a direct no is super uncomfortable or comes across as rude, you can say, "No, thank you," politely and firmly. Pay attention to how many times you say yes when you really mean no. In order to create loving boundaries for yourself and others, it's essential you learn these skills. Say no to anything that doesn't add value to your life or makes you feel uncomfortable. Trust your intuition and gut feeling on things. Saying no in this way takes the pressure away from you. It prevents you worrying about the same questions reoccurring. For example, take the question, would you like to come out tonight? In my old people-pleasing ways, I may have said, "I'm so sorry. I've got a ton of work to do and then I need to visit my parents." A full, elongated story. The real reason may be that I actually don't want to go out with this person. Unless we give a direct no, this person will ask again. They are not doing it to be annoying or put pressure on you. They are totally unaware that you actually don't want to go out with them. Short-term pain, my lovely, for long-term gain. You can do it.

Set Some Boundaries

For me, I love a full diary, meeting friends, catching up etc. But often this can leave me feeling overwhelmed. There are some things in my diary now that are set. It would take something huge and amazingly exciting to knock them out. My yoga and meditation are scheduled. For me these are essential to my mental health, as is my bedtime. During the week, I'm in bed by 9 p.m., lights out 9.30, as I'm generally up at 5.30. I've discovered that this is what works for me and has me feeling at my best. I'm not saying I never 100 per cent deviate from this, but I have set these boundaries so it's easier for me to say no to going out in the evenings.

Workwise, I've discovered that I can only say yes to doing one totally new event or project a week. If I commit to delivering two completely new things in the same week, I get super anxious, overwhelmed, and stressed. It's not pleasant for me or my family.

My calendar is now my new best friend. Initially, I thought scheduling all my activities was a bit OCD and really overwhelming. It was only overwhelming, however, because it forced me to look at my life on a daily basis and see how overcommitted I was. It made me realise that the to do-list I had for each day was physically impossible to achieve timewise. Learn to love your schedule.

Exercise 4: It's time to get real with your diary. You can use an electronic calendar or a paper diary, whichever you prefer. I lurve a paper diary, and it has taken me some time to embrace my electronic one. But now it keeps me sane. You can then repeat recurring events, get alarms, and see your week really clearly. If using a paper one, you will need to have each hour broken down. At first, it may appear a little crazy and so much to fill in. But you will begin to see just how all your yessing is leaving you overcommitted. Schedule everything in your calendar. Schedule food shopping, cleaning, work, meeting friends, reading, hobbies, family time, going to the gym, appointments, correspondence time, lunch, dinner, eating and prep, menu planning, weekly review, and next week's calendar scheduling. Even wake up and bedtimes to ensure you get the sleep you need for your body. Set yourself realistic times for each.

I'd suggest if using your electronic calendar that you colour code your events or pop them into categories: work, family time, friends, self-care, leisure, and so on. That way, you will easily see at a glance how much time you are spending in each and where the imbalance lies.

So looking at your calendar now, how much free time and freedom do you have? I'm guessing not so much. Now look at your calendar and see what things make you feel yucky or fill you with dread. What's taking up most of your time? What can you instantly remove? Are there things there that you have overcommitted to? Can you stop them? If you can't stop them, can you reschedule them to another week, month, year? Are there things you'd love to be doing but feel you have no space to do them? Things like reading a book or taking a bath.

To begin with, you need to schedule all activities. This will make them happen. Scheduling your self-care is a priority. Scheduling will make it more likely to take place. Your health, well-being, and love for yourself are important. Scheduling will help prevent you from being so impulsive with your saying yes to things that don't support you. It will enable you to identify any periods of time where you may be overstretched or busy. You can then act upon making changes, looking for support, ensuring you have something healthy in for dinner those nights. Although planning may seem boring or restrictive, it actually allows the opposite. It gives you back control, returns your power, and allows you to be in charge of your life. It allows you to release anxiety as you can clearly see in a day what you'd like to achieve.

Your calendar will go from being overwhelming to being your friend and a great tool to help you create the loving boundaries you require to live the life you desire.

Now is the time for you to go forth and show others how you wish to be treated. Be strong. Unless we clearly set out how we wish to be treated and how we wish to spend our time, we will continuously be stuck in the cycle of compromising our own needs and potentially being treated unfairly. Release the fear. People will not love you any less by you saying no. If they do, it is a sure-fire example of them having taken advantage of your people-pleasing ways in the past.

It's time to take your time back. Setting boundaries and saying no will create time and space to do the things you love and be with those you love. When the world is such a demanding and busy place, you need to take control. You'll no longer say you're too busy or feel compromised because your life will be focused on the things you love. You will be making conscious choices and decisions. Decisions that support you. Your mental, physical, and spiritual health will all be supported. If you master this one chapter, I can assure you that your life will change. Your anxiety will drop, you won't be overwhelmed, and you'll feel more joyful, vibrant, and empowered. I've got your back. You can do this.

In the long run, we shape our lives, and we shape ourselves. The process never ends until we die. And the choices we make are ultimately our responsibility.
—Eleanor Roosevelt

Notes page

Chapter 4
Feeding Freedom: Food and Nutrition: The Dos and Don'ts of Living a Vibrant Life

I nourish my body with healthy food;
my body sparkles with vitality.

This chapter will change your life. If you implement just some of these suggestions, your anxiety will improve. This is not a quick-fix diet; this is a lifestyle, a lifestyle you will love and flourish in. Your body and mind will thank you, your self-love will grow, and your gratitude and love for the amazing machine that is your body will develop.

Oh, how food can be my nemesis and saviour. I grew up a cake-loving, carb-craving sugar addict. I would eat condensed milk from the tin with a spoon. When the panic attacks started when I was 15, not once did the doctor mention that my diet or the fact that my teenage hormones were developing had anything to do with them. As time went on, I noticed how my anxiety and panic would grow around hormonal time. At 16, my diet consisted of microwave pizzas, Pepsi, and crisps. This was by no means suitable for fuelling my developing and active body. I loved horses and worked at a local stable. I would cycle there, muck out stables, and ride horses; during this time, I'd get through the day eating chocolate and pot noodles. As I got older and began to drink alcohol, the panic would increase like a beast taking over my nights out. The next day, I would be consumed by fear, anxiety, and guilt. Add in some caffeine in the form of Red Bull or cola, and you have the perfect diet for giving you anxiety.

As time moved on, the self-loathing and desire to fit in began. I would try fad diets: Slim Fast, cabbage soup, Dr Atkins, counting calories, diet pills, and patches. My anxiety would grow like a volcano waiting to erupt, as my body screamed at me to stop and listen. Anxiety isn't there to make your life hell; it's there to help you tune in and listen to what has become imbalanced.

"Anxiety isn't there to make your life hell; it is there to help you tune in and listen to what has become imbalanced."

In my late teens and university years, as I began to party, my diet was horrendous. I consumed more caffeine to help me focus, stay up later, and get through uni. I would take pro plus and guarana to give me that buzz. My body began to fail me; I developed psoriasis. It started in small patches on my arms and elbows, and then it, like the anxiety I was experiencing, grew. It began to cover my whole body. My body was flaky, and my life felt flaky. My self-confidence plummeted. My mind told me I was unattractive, that people would look at me and be disgusted. I had to wear clothes that covered my body fully, to hide the signs of stress and abuse I had put my body through. I got various creams and tablets from the doctor, and again not once was my diet mentioned. To control the anxiety and panic, my doctor prescribed beta blockers and suggested antidepressants. Even in my teens, I didn't feel this was the right route for me. I have a vague recollection of taking the beta blockers, but even then, I was anxious taking them.

My parents could see how much I was struggling with my skin, and in their bid to remove my pain, my dad found a magic potion online, some interesting, natural collection of herbs, plants, and creams. This helped clear and soothe my skin. The flare-ups would still happen occasionally, but this natural miracle was my saviour.

The NHS state that "psoriasis is a long-lasting

(chronic) disease that usually involves periods when you have no symptoms or mild symptoms, followed by periods when symptoms are more severe. There's no cure for psoriasis, but a range of treatments can improve symptoms and the appearance of skin patches." The Psoriasis Society also states the same: "There is no cure." I can categorically state that for me, there was a cure, and it wasn't chemical-laden creams. It was reducing stress and improving my lifestyle.

Through the end of my teenage years and into adulthood, food was my emotional crutch (it still is). If I'm happy, I would celebrate with cake; if I was sad, I would celebrate with cake. If I experienced success or failure or rejection? Yep, you guessed it: cake. At one point, I was sales and marketing manager for a multimillion-pound bakery in charge of new product development and sales of cake (this was actually one of my favourite jobs, surprise, surprise). The irony isn't lost on me.

I loved everything about food: creating, making, eating. I started my own catering business, but the pressure caused me to return to my self-destructing ways. Late nights, early mornings, alcohol, sugar, and caffeine. Bam, let the breakdown commence. My relationships broke down, my self-worth broke down, and then my business broke down. I remember sitting on the back steps of my friend's bar, breathing into a brown bag, hyperventilating, lips numb as I struggled to breathe through my panic attack.

Looking back, it's easy to see now the cycle and the links between food and anxiety, but when you're in it, you're trying to survive.

I don't want you to go through the same cycles that I did. If you already are, I hope that this chapter can throw you a lifeline.

In my early thirties, after giving birth to my daughter, the solution seeking commenced fully. I'd been to the hospital for scans, I'd attended CBT, I was never away from the doctor. The panic attacks had developed into me feeling like I was going to black out. In another bid to support and help me, my parents suggested I see a natural medicine practitioner. As I sat in her chair, I cried when we went over my list of symptoms. I suddenly felt understood. She pulled a book from her shelf and showed me a condition called adrenal fatigue. The symptoms in the book and the symptoms in my list matched. Relief flooded my body. I wasn't mad; the symptoms I was experiencing were those of this condition, and there was a way out.

I immediately started a recovery plan. Key to this plan was diet. Being a new mum and mum of three, my diet consisted of quick, easy food. Lots of pasta, glasses of wine, and caffeine. Surprisingly, this current diet was not supporting or nourishing my body, and it certainly wasn't going to give me the vibrant and healthy life I yearned for.

My natural medicine practitioner educated me in nutritional support and showed me how to use my food to benefit my health. I began to see food as fuel. What I put in was what I got out. If I put in fast food for a quick fix, it would be exactly that. If I put in nutrient dense food, high in antioxidants, my body would function and thrive.

In this chapter, I'll highlight the foods that support and nourish your body as well as those to avoid.

Let food be thy medicine and medicine be thy food.
—Hippocrates

This is seriously simple and common sense. However, as I've said previously, it may not be easy. But it's so worth it. What you will achieve is a sustainable lifestyle, a lifestyle and diet that will support you daily, through life's periods of stress and joy. Are you ready?

First off, I am not a nutritionist, doctor, or naturopath. I am an anxiety sufferer who has spent the past two decades researching and trying to find a solution. This information is based on my own experience, research papers, my own visits to professional nutritionists, doctors, natural medicine practitioners, trial and error, and lots and lots of reading. These key areas are the ones I have found to make the most impact in my own journey to overcome anxiety.

These are the biggest impact makers when using food for support:

- healthy blood sugar levels
- balancing hormones
- reducing synthetics and fake food
- reducing stimulants and inflammatory foods
- increasing nutrients
- hydration

All of this can be achieved through eating real food and some awesome nutritional supplementation. This can be so much fun, and you will see results quickly in your mood, emotions, and overall health.

Let's begin.

Healthy Blood Sugar Levels

What does this even mean? As I got to know myself and better understood my responses to anxiety, although I thought there wasn't a particular trigger, I became aware that there were periods when my anxiety was so much worse. What I discovered was if I was hungry or had pigged out, drunk loads of sugary drinks and alcohol, my anxiety went through the roof.

If I ate little and often, my anxiety was more in check. So why was this? When we consume sugary or food that has a high glycaemic load, it causes peaks in our blood sugars. The more dramatic the response your body has to blood sugar, the more insulin your body needs to release in order to bring your blood sugars back to a healthy level. High blood sugar levels put stress on the body. The body then releases cortisol. Cortisol is also known as the stress hormone. We'll find out more about this in the section on balancing hormones.

So how do we prevent these huge peaks and troughs in blood sugars?

1: We eat regularly and have healthy snacks.
2: We limit processed foods.
3: We reduce refined-sugar cakes, chocolate, white pastas.
4: We eat food that are low GI (Glycaemic Index).

The Glycaemic Index is a way of ranking foods based on their effect on blood sugars. When we eat foods that are low GI, this creates a more stable effect on blood sugars. Allowing you to feel fuller for longer and prevents the huge highs and lows you can feel mood wise from the increase or drop in blood sugar levels. You've heard the phrase "Hangry"? When your mood is so crazy mad because you just need some food. The *Oxford Dictionary* even now recognises this word. "Hangry: Bad-tempered or irritable as a result of hunger." This is what you want to avoid. This happens because your blood sugar level has dropped.

Here are some examples of what to eat and what to avoid. These will help you thrive and bring balance:

- Fruits, including apples, berries, grapes, pears
- Vegetables, including peppers, spinach, aubergine, tomatoes, onions, broccoli, cauliflower
- Dairy: eggs, cheese, unsweetened yogurt
- Protein: legumes, nuts, seeds, beans, avocado's, lentils, oatmeal, lean meat, fish, turkey, chicken, salmon, haddock
- Grains: Brown rice and pasta, quinoa, whole-wheat bread

Then I love using nut butters, hummus, olive or avocado oils, tamari, and lots of herbs and spices. As a vegetarian, I really have to make sure I'm getting enough protein in my diet from plant sources, so I love snacking on nuts and homemade energy balls.

High-GI: These will cause you to get a blood sugar high, followed by a crash. I'm not saying never eat these; far from it. I'm all for balance and eating what works for you as an individual. I would try to keep these to a minimum or as treats in your diet:

- Fruits: pineapple, kiwi, dates
- Vegetables: potatoes, carrots
- Dairy: ice cream, sweetened yoghurt, and milk shakes
- Meat: Meat does not cause spikes in your blood sugars as such, but too much meat may lead to inflammation in the body, so it's worth having in moderation.
- Grains: white bread, bagels, couscous, white rice

Lots of processed foods will be high GI due to the added sugars, like doughnuts and pastries and pizza. Lots of packaged snacks can be full of hidden sugars too, so limit them too.

Regular balanced meals and snacks are what we should do; this will help us feel more balanced and be less irritable and anxious throughout the day.

Balancing Hormones

Our hormones can make us do things, say things, and behave in some crazy ways if they're unbalanced. I used to be a full-blown she-wolf. Stress really affects our hormones as does diet, sleep, weight, underlying health conditions, birth control, toxins, and chemicals. It is suggested that 80 per cent of women will experience hormone imbalance at some point in their lives. It's a growing issue with rising infertility rates and more hormone-related illnesses.

How do you know if you're experiencing hormone imbalance?

Signs of imbalance:

- ✓ fatigue
- ✓ weight gain
- ✓ night sweats
- ✓ anxiety
- ✓ depression
- ✓ low libido
- ✓ weight gain or loss
- ✓ hair loss
- ✓ acne
- ✓ blurred vision
- ✓ tender breasts

- ✓ memory fog
- ✓ headaches and migraine
- ✓ infertility

The above list looked like a mirror. I was experiencing it all, bar the acne and hair loss (silver lining). My hormone imbalance was eventually diagnosed when I was 30. I had been working out hard, eating right, and the weight just wasn't shifting. We were trying for a baby, and nothing was happening. We were told we could never conceive naturally, then bam, it happened. My baby miracle was conceived in 2009. It wasn't until I conceived that the doctors picked up I had an underlying thyroid condition.

Let's rewind a moment and learn a little about hormones and the body, and you'll understand why an imbalance in this area can cause anxiety, stress, and low mood. I'm going to keep the science to a minimum, as this book isn't a medical journal. It's a lifestyle guide written from one anxiety sufferer to another. I want to cut through the wordiness and science and just tell you how to get better and lead a life beyond your wildest dreams.

But first, just a teeny, tiny bit of science.

Hormones are created by our endocrine system. Endocrine glands include the thyroid, adrenal, penial, pituitary, thymus, ovaries, and testes. The main hormones we're going to look at are serotonin and cortisol.

We're looking to boost our serotonin and reduce or cortisol. Serotonin is often referred to as the happy hormone and cortisol as the stress hormone.

Let's start with serotonin, the happy hormone. Although serotonin is produced in our brain, 90 per cent of it can be found in our gut and digestive tract. This why food has such a huge impact on our serotonin production and levels. Serotonin plays a crucial role in communication between our brains and bodies for all sorts of things. It's like a little messenger travelling round our bodies, delivering information. When production is low, communication to our brain is reduced, and this can play havoc with our mood, emotions, sleep, memory, and learnings.

WebMD states, "There are many researchers who believe that an imbalance in serotonin levels may influence mood in a way that leads to depression. Possible problems include low brain cell production of serotonin, a lack of receptor sites able to receive the serotonin that is made, inability of serotonin to reach the receptor sites, or a shortage in tryptophan, the chemical from which serotonin is made. If any of these biochemical glitches occur, researchers believe it can lead to depression, as well as obsessive-compulsive disorder, anxiety, panic, and even excess anger."

This is why many people are prescribed antidepressants that are serotonin based.

What if we could improve our serotonin naturally? Well, we can. Here's a list of serotonin-boosting foods. The foods we're going to look at all contain one key chemical: an amino acid called tryptophan. Tryptophan is a chemical that the body requires to synthesise serotonin. The key to using this as a way of boosting serotonin is to accompany tryptophan-rich food with a heathy carb.

Tryptophan-rich foods include eggs, cheese, turkey, salmon, nuts and seeds, tofu, oats, beans, avocado, lentils, and pineapples. And wait for it ... chocolate. Yes, chocolate. Woooo hoooo. We're looking for cacao-rich chocolate. So lots of similarities to the low-GI foods mentioned previously.

In addition to this, I highly recommend a good pro- and prebiotic to support healthy gut bacteria, making your guts a healthy environment for serotonin.

Other nonfood ways to boost our serotonin levels include getting outside and gaining some sunlight on our skin, exercising, smiling, and as a little mood-boosting treat, a massage. I get a massage once a month and schedule it as one of my self-care essentials.

Reducing Cortisol

When we have too much cortisol, this can lead to adrenal fatigue. Having suffered from this, I can testify it's incredibly debilitating. Stress coursing through your body affects your sleep. Cortisol is an essential hormone. It helps support our blood sugars, regulates salt and water intake, works as an anti-inflammatory, and influences blood pressure. Too much cortisol, however, has been shown to increase depression, anxiety, mood swings, and fatigue.

If you feel your cortisol may be high, it probably is, if you experience anxiety or ongoing stress for any length of time. Functioning at a high level of stress on a daily basis will cause your cortisol to go through the roof and place additional pressure on your adrenals. It's all a vicious circle, but one we can escape from. You can get your cortisol levels checked. This is a simple test you can do using your saliva. I advise my clients to do this, as it's a great visual to check back and see how you've managed to reduce stress. You can find further details of this on my website. Testing is a great way to monitor your health and give you a clue as to what's going on in your body internally. You don't need to test in order for the following to help.

Cortisol-Reducing Foods

- ✓ dark chocolate
- ✓ bananas and pears
- ✓ black or green tea
- ✓ blueberries
- ✓ probiotics
- ✓ vitamin C-containing foods such as oranges
- ✓ soya beans
- ✓ healthy oils: avocado, coconut
- ✓ flaxseeds (these are also great for hormonal balance)

These are your go-to munchies to help reduce stress from cortisol.

Other ways to support your hormone balance is ensuring you get enough good quality sleep, maintaining a healthy body weight, drinking water, and staying hydrated. Exercise is also critical.

Reducing Synthetics and Fake Food

Keep it real, and keep it clean.

Our body is the most incredible machine; the more you learn, the more it blows your mind. When we think of our body as a machine, it's almost easier to think about how to fuel it. What we put in, we get out. If you put diesel in a petrol car, it's going to break. Not immediately, but slowly, the diesel will damage the engine and fuel system. The same is true for our bodies. If we add fake food and synthetics, our body will slowly begin to break. Our body is so incredibly clever; it will tolerate so much. It really does want to be our friend. It's our job to maintain this friendship.

What do I mean by synthetics and fake food? I mean anything that is produced in a lab; we're talking anything that doesn't come from nature: synthetic and artificial sweeteners, preservatives, and other chemical compounds. In today's food market, it's difficult to avoid all synthetics but if you're eating wholefoods, fresh and homemade, you're off to a great start. Why is this important? Our body has been created to use wholefoods, not processed, chemical-laden foods. Eating these foods can lead to a build-up in toxins and nutritional imbalances. Our body needs us to make educated decisions. When we add toxins to our body, it increases the stress on an already stressed and inflamed system.

Reducing Stimulants and Inflammatory Foods

When we are stressed, our body is already in a heightened state. Yes, we may be absolutely exhausted, but our body is ready to jump into action and let fear arise at any given moment. The fatigue takes control, and we want to reach for that caffeine-laden drink or sugary hit to get us through. Caffeine will have the same effect as the blood sugar highs and lows we spoke of earlier.

If you're addicted to Starbucks or need that morning coffee to kick-start your day, it's time for them to go. Hasta la vista, caffeine. I don't know how many clients I have who come to me with anxiety, and they rely so heavily on caffeine. Attributing the heart palpitations, clammy hands, and jittery feelings to anxiety, when actually, their Starbucks and Red Bull addictions are sending their heart racing and having them feeling in a spin. Caffeine-like anxiety stimulates our fight-or-flight response. It can actually trigger an anxiety attack. It can leave you nervous and moody, and disrupt your sleep. Caffeine can hide in other places than our coffee. I used to take guarana supplements, weight loss supplements, and even some cold and flu over-the-counter medicines that had caffeine.

Exercise 1: Kick the caffeine; it needs to go. We're so lucky that today, there is pretty much decaf everything. Embrace the herbal teas and decaf americanos. No halfways; it just has to go. Buzz off, caffeine.

Inflammation is something quite different. Inflammation is the body's response to a threat. This can be seen when you bash your knee, and it swells and bruises, or when you catch a virus, and your body gets all systems go to fight it off. When we are in the inflammatory state, our bodies have to work super hard. By reducing inflammation, we remove and alleviate some of the pressure.

The foods we eat can trigger an inflammatory response; coupled with stress and anxiety, this puts our beautiful bodies under so much pressure. Author and head of psychiatry at the University of Cambridge, Edward Bullmore, states, "Inflammation in your body could be a factor causing depression." Dr Vincent Pedre explains, "Inflammation causes oxidative stress (a form of biological stress), which leads to distress signals in the brain that can lead to either depression or anxiety-or both." The science and proof are there so what do we need to. We need to avoid inflammatory foods and increase anti-inflammatory foods. Let's get more of those antioxidant and super foods.

Inflammatory Foods to Avoid

processed meats
sugary drinks
white bread
gluten
processed snacks such as crisps
alcohol
ice cream and biscuits
margarine

Some people find tomatoes, potatoes, and peppers can also trigger an inflammatory response.

Anti-Inflammatory Foods

My number one is curcumin, otherwise known as turmeric. This really is a super food and one I highly suggest you add to your diet. I share my turmeric paste recipe below. I take a teaspoon in the morning and a teaspoon at night in some warm nut milk, with a teaspoon of manuka honey and a sprinkle of cinnamon. It makes the perfect turmeric latte, and it's lush.

olive oil
blueberries, strawberries, raspberries, cherries, oranges

oily fish including salmon, mackerel, sardines
broccoli
avocados
peppers
mushrooms
grapes
dark choc and cacao
almonds, walnuts
green leafy veggies, spinach, and kale

Hydration

Go grab a glass of water and get ready to rehydrate. I don't know about you, but if I don't drink a lot of water, it affects my anxiety, stress levels, and mood. Our body relies heavily on water to function correctly. When we become dehydrated, we become stressed and release cortisol, which then puts our body into an alert state. Increased cortisol and reduced hydration can cause headaches, muscle weakness, lethargy, heart palpitations, and difficulty concentrating and focusing. It can also leave you feeling foggy-brained. So this was enough for me to feel anxious. Previously, when my body was like this, I usually had a panic attack too.

So simply ensuring we get enough water can calm our system and help our bodies operate at optimum level. In the UK, the NHS recommends drinking six to eight glasses of water a day. This is around 1.3 litres. In the United States, it is advised to drink eight glasses a day, around 1.9 litres. I'd aim for the US target of around 1.9 litres of water. This doesn't just meet our basic core functioning needs but also has additional health benefits. If you live where it's hot, you will need to account for this, so definitely go to the higher range of the two options.

I have a reusable water bottle I use daily; this makes it a lot easier to keep track of what I am drinking. I know if I haven't had enough water, I feel really moody and grumpy, and I struggle to concentrate and focus. Excuse to go treat yourself to a funky water bottle.

Do you notice your anxiety is worse after a night drinking alcohol? Alcohol dehydrates the body, affects blood sugar, and causes inflammation. So although it may be fun at the time, the effect on your body after is not great. Alcohol, being a depressant, will really not support your mood. Alcohol even effects the serotonin in your body, so it can lead to greater anxiety and depression. Alcohol used to be a go-to for me, especially in social situations. It's actually suggested that 20 per cent of social anxiety sufferers have alcohol-dependency issues. I totally get that, as it was a way to release anxiety and get that Dutch courage.

Now I am completely alcohol free, not because I was addicted but because I couldn't cope any more with the anxiety that followed the drinking; some call it beer fear. It's hugely common for anxiety to follow an episode of drinking; for some, this may only last a few hours. For others, it can be a whole day. This was the point I got to, and for me, it just wasn't worth it any more.

If you feel you may have issues with alcohol dependence, it's advisable to chat this through with your doctor. There are so many wonderful support systems in place.

> Take care of your body. It's the
> only place you have to live.
> —Jim Rohn

You now know the great and not-so-great choices; now it's time to put them into practice. Let's do this.

Exercise 2: Keep a food diary for a week. In this diary, record absolutely everything you eat or drink. At this stage, I am not asking you to make any changes. I'm just looking for you to bring awareness to your current eating and drinking habits. If you have any great days where you feel anxiety free, or if your anxiety is bad on a particular day, make a note of this too. Bringing awareness to current behaviours gives you the opportunity to make supportive and lasting changes. You can download a food diary tool at www. spiritandsoul.me.

OK, let's get this anxiety-bashing and mood-boosting menu on the go. These are my go-to meals to keep my brain and body working together for a happy, healthy mood. I'm pescatarian, but you could easily have the same but pop in some turkey or any other lean meat.

Breakfast

- Green smoothie with avocado, peanut butter, banana, spinach, cinnamon, and any plant-based milk. Chuck it all in the blender, and mix until smooth. Sometimes, I'll add a shot of protein or a handful of cashews if I know I've got a busy day or a yoga class ahead.
- Overnight oats: this is one of my daughter's faves, and it makes breakfast a cinch: 1 cup gluten-free rolled oats, 1 tablespoon chia seeds, 1 cup of milk (I love rice or coconut), 1 tablespoon maple syrup. Combine all ingredients in a bowl and mix. Pop into glass jar, refrigerate overnight, and boom: breakfast all ready and good to go in the

morning. Sometimes, we pop fresh blueberries on top.

- Porridge made with oat or nut milk, topped with berries and seeds, sweetened with natural sweetener such as maple syrup.

Lunch

- Gluten-free oatcakes with cheese or hummus
- Vegetable-packed soup or lentil soup (I pack in the vitamins and feed my body)
- Poached eggs on gluten-free toast, with spinach and black pepper

Dinner

- Cashew stir-fry: load up your wok with as much colour and veggies as you can, add cashews, tofu, salmon, or turkey for a super yummy, quick, and nutritious dinner.
- Omelettes and salad. There's a whole lot of eggs get munched in our home; we're super lucky that we have Betty, Bluebell, and Becky supplying us with organic free-range eggs daily. You can mix up all the fillings you like. I love black olives, spinach, and goat cheese.
- Quinoa vegetable chilli with avocado

Snacks

Fruit, nuts, seeds, hummus and crudities, hard-boiled eggs, energy balls, some dark chocolate, turmeric latte.

My go-to suggestions are merely that—suggestions; you can create your own menu. It's great to have a list on hand for the days when you're stuck and likely to grab processed or sugar-laden foods. This part can be so much fun. Trying new things and feeling how food can affect your mood. You'll feel vibrant, alert, and more connected to your body.

Exercise 3: Write your food plan weekly. Start today. Planning your meals in advance not only encourages you to make positive choices; it also reduces decision fatigue when you're super tired, cuts your food bill, and generates less food waste. Win-win. You can download the Be Free Weekly Food Planner Tool at www.spiritandsoul.me.

Increasing Nutrients and Supplementation

With the best will and diet in the world, you may still be missing vital nutrients. The over farming and overproduction of our soils means that our food no longer contains the same quantity and quality of nutrients. Every day, I take a multivitamin, omega oils, and pro- and prebiotics.

I advise you to source a natural and high-quality multivitamin. You can find them online or in your local health food store. They need to come from a natural source, or your body won't know how to use them.

Next up: gut health. Probiotics and prebiotics are a great way to support our guts from undue stress and imbalance. Probiotics are yeasts and bacteria that are good for your gut health, returning the previously stressed gut to a healthy, happy balanced area. With so many studies linking gut health and brain health, this is an area worth implementing. Prebiotics are basically the food for the probiotics. This allows the good bacteria to grow and build in the gut.

Omega-3 oils are the final nutritional supplement I take daily. I first noticed a significant difference to mental health when my son started using omega oils to support his concentration and Asperger's. I not only noticed the improvement in his behaviour, but his eyes were brighter, and he was more connected. Why I didn't think all those years back that I could take them myself, I don't know.

Our diets tend to contain more omega-6 than omega-3. For the body and mind to work efficiently, there needs to be a 50/50 balance of these fats. Omega-3 actually calms inflammation in the body and supports hormone health. Omega-6, on the other hand, promotes inflammation in the body. Omega-3 comes in the form of oily fish, such as salmon and mackerel, hempseeds, walnuts, flaxseeds, avocado, and chia seeds. Omega-6 is polyunsaturated fat. These are increasing in our modern-day diet due to them being used in processed foods, meats, cured meats, cakes, and margarines. A diet high in omega-6 has now been linked to coronary issues and even some cancers. Balance, as with all foody choices, is key.

On the plus side, supplementation of omega-3 oils is simple. Research has shown that supplementing your diet with omega-3 can lower blood pressure, decrease risk of heart attack and stroke, and improve brain health and cognitive function. I find this area most important to me and for the purposes of this book. Supplementation of omega-3 has been shown to decrease depression and anxiety. Studies have also shown ADHD, schizophrenia, bipolar, dementia, and other mental illness can all be supported with omega-3 supplementation. This natural oil is an amazing tool to add to your overcoming anxiety food toolkit.

Exercise 4: Purchase the following and add them into your daily diet. Feel your body vibrate as it receives the nutrients and support it requires to function efficiently. High-vibe life, here you come.

- ✓ probiotics
- ✓ multivitamins
- ✓ omega oils

Not all nutritional supplements are created equal; many contain synthetics and fillers, so seek advice from a reliable source or and read the label. If you don't know what the ingredients are on the label, don't buy it.

Summary

This chapter offers common-sense diet and food advice. This type of eating is so simple. Yes, it takes willpower to not reach for that cake or large latte to get you through, but when you think about food as fuel, and see that what we put in is what we get out, it makes it easy. You will feel greater clarity, your body will feel calmer, you will feel loved, and you'll become your own best friend instead of something you resent.

Small steps daily will deliver huge results, and the absolute bonus is, you're going to feel great along the way.

If you're struggling on your own, it can be super helpful to visit a professional to get you started on the right path. There are a number of natural medicine practitioners, nutritionists, and naturopaths who can support you on this journey.

Good luck, my lovely; you got this.

Notes page

Chapter 5
The Great Outdoors

I feel connected, strong, and safe.

When I was at my lowest and my balance was all over the place, the last thing I wanted to do was step outside. It was the fear of being seen, fear of being outside my safety and comfort zone, fear I would have a panic attack and be unable to get home. Yet every time I did go for a walk or visit my horses, I felt better. Why was this?

I have come to discover that being outside in nature is a hugely important part of recovery from anxiety, stress, and depression. Not only are you breathing in fresh air, but you are aligning with and grounding yourself with the earth's energy.

As we go through daily life, we pick up positive energy charges, disrupting our balance; the earth's charge is negative, so when we come into contact with it, it actually helps neutralise us and balance our energy.

Sounds pretty cosmic, doesn't it? However, it has been scientifically shown that earthing, or grounding using the earth's neutralising properties, has huge health benefits. In today's modern society, we are increasingly exposed to things which disrupt us energetically. This could be your mobile phone, laptop, TV, electricity cables—anything that emits electromagnetic frequencies. A summary published in the *Journal of Environmental and Public Health* states, "Grounding appears to improve sleep, normalize the day–night cortisol rhythm, reduce pain, reduce stress, shift the autonomic nervous system from sympathetic toward parasympathetic activation, increase heart rate variability, speed wound healing, and reduce blood viscosity."

What does it all mean? The science part, according to Dr John Briffa, author of *Ultimate Health,* is that "during the normal processes of metabolism the body generates what are called 'reactive oxygen species' which are commonly referred to as 'free radicals.' These compounds appear to be important, at least in part because they have the ability to attack and destroy unwanted things within the body, including bacteria and viruses. However, too many free radicals are a bad thing and have been implicated in chronic disease and well as the very process of ageing.

"Free radicals are involved in the process known

as inflammation, which is part of the healing process. However, low-grade inflammation throughout the body may lead to pain and other problems In the muscles and joints and is also believed to be a key driving factor in many chronic diseases including heart disease and type 2 diabetes. In short, we want free radicals, but not too many.

"Free radicals lack sparks of energy known as 'electrons.' One way to quell them is to give them electrons, and these can be supplied by nutrients such as vitamins A, C and E, and plant substances known as 'polyphenols' (found in, among other things, tea, coffee, cocoa and apples). However, substances we eat and drink are not the only way to get electrons into the body: earthing does this too. If the body has a positive charge on it, earthing allows electrons to flow into the body where, in theory, they can neutralize overblown free radical and inflammatory damage.

"Carrying a positive charge may well affect the body in lots of different ways, which means that earthing may offer a range of wellbeing benefits."

How do we ground ourselves? What does that even mean? I remember thinking that's so hippy-dippy, grounding: "Oh, I'm feeling so ungrounded." Now, I realise that when we are stressed or anxious, it is actually a necessity and an essential part of living a healthy and relaxed life.

So how do you know if you're ungrounded? Do you ever get that feeling of being a bit all in your head or spacey, just not fully connected with what's happening around you? Are you overly emotional? Do you feel like life is happening and you're not quite part of it? Or really fearful and not sure why? That knot in your gut and your heart is racing? For me, I would literally feel unbalanced. I would feel wobbly, unstable, anxious, and scared. This is when I would need to be grounded.

"To be connected to the earth is to be connected to our self, our soul, our life: rooted, safe, and secure."

When you're on holiday and did your feet in the sand and sea, breathing in that beautiful sea air, and you get that feeling of *Ahhh, I wish I could feel like this every day*. Yes, it could be because you're away from home and have fewer cares, but did you know you were actually grounding yourself at the same time? Water and sand are actually conductors of the earth's energy; they will assist in the grounding and balancing process. So walking barefoot, even standing barefoot in your garden, can help you connect and ground yourself.

Pretty awesome stuff. But maybe you're saying,

"Susi, where I live, it's freezing cold," or "I live in a city, nowhere near a beach. I'm not about to go barefoot in the sand." Have no fear, there are other solutions (although I regularly dip my toes in the North Sea of Scotland and walk barefoot on the icy sand).

Grounding Exercise 1: Take off your socks and shoes. Find a grassy spot (or beach, if you're lucky enough to have one close at hand). Plant your feet firmly on the ground. Roll your shoulders back, spine straight, crown of the head reaching up towards the sky. If you feel comfortable, allow your eyes to gently close. Take in a deep breath through your nose, feeling your chest rise and your tummy expand, and then exhale slowly. Repeat the deep breath in, but this time, I want you to imagine the outbreath is travelling down and into the earth below you through your feet; do this three times. Then lastly, imagine as you breathe in that you are drawing the breath up from the feet, through the earth, and then pushing the outbreath back down through the body, right down to the soles of the feet and into the ground beneath. Do this three times. Now stop, allow your breath to fall into its natural rhythm, and just make a mental note of how you now feel. Do you feel more relaxed? Do you feel more connected?

As a side note, if you are unable to leave the house,

this can be done standing or seated in a chair with your bare feet planted on the floor. If this is the case, you can visualise the beach or grass. Really engage with the sensations. How do you think this would feel? Use the breath in the same way as above.

Being outside allows us to connect with nature and align ourselves to the earth's rhythms, notice the changing seasons, and appreciate the beauty around us. It allows us to realise we are part of something greater than our own immediate reality. When we are by ourselves, in our own homes, it is easy to disconnect from the world. Our world seems smaller, and our problems seem larger. Getting outside offers a fresh perspective, a chance to breathe fresh air and get new ideas. If you struggle to leave home, see if you can find a friend or family member to support you. It can be for a five-minute walk round the block. The important thing is that you set yourself small achievable goals and build from there. You are attempting to reduce the stress and anxiety on your body, so keep it simple, achievable, and something that isn't going to put you into fight-or-flight response.

Getting outside for me initially was a challenge, especially since it was a busy environment. I used to think, *Just get over it; put yourself out there. Stop being so stupid.* But in actual fact, I was doing more harm than good by this constant pressure. I was causing my body to release stress hormones and increasing my negative experiences. You want to keep it simple, a little challenging but achievable. Then you can slowly and steadily build upon your experience.

Anything that connects you with the earth's energy will help with grounding, so gardening is a great way to connect. Don't have a garden? You could always volunteer with a local community group (so much value doing something like this socially, from making a contribution and from a grounding point of view), seek an allotment, or just buy some potted plants for your home.

Plants can have other positive effects for your home. Rosemary, for example, promotes physical and mental health whilst cleansing and purifying the air. This can also reduce the toxic load in your home. From an aromatherapy point of view, rosemary can lift your mood, reduce tiredness, decrease anxious feelings, improve memory, and help insomnia. Rosemary is also said to bring inner peace. Bliss, grounding, and uplifting: double-win. Aloe vera and orchids are said to bring positive energy. You can have fun with it. Bring life, love, and energy into your home whilst getting your fingernails dirty and connecting with nature.

You can buy equipment to help with grounding, such

as mats, special shoes, and patches. I own a grounding mat and find it beneficial, but ultimately, there are many natural and inexpensive solutions you can use.

Visiting a forest or a park with trees is another wonderful way to connect with this beautiful grounding energy. Being around trees has been shown to reduce symptoms of depression and anxiety. There's something so truly calming about trees. We can gather great strength and learning from trees.

Case Study: Elaine. Elaine is 40; she was working full-time in a stressful job. She also looked after her family, two boys and her hubbie, and crammed in as much as she could socially. She got up before her kids did to squeeze in an hour's work before breakfast. In her words, she was just functioning through life. Elaine first came to me purely out of curiosity to try meditation. I worked near her home, so she thought she would give it a try. She booked a block of meditation and decided to make a commitment to herself.

Elaine and her family were always very active and sporty; they regularly spent time outdoors, but this relationship with the great outdoors was a way to grow.

The interesting thing about Elaine, and for so many of us, is that we think we're fine. We are coping, functioning, and the lives we are leading are totally normal—as is the stress we endure daily. We put up with negativity around us; we head into a negative work environment, where we sit surrounded by It on a daily basis. Here's the wonderful thing: once we start exploring meditation or self-development, our minds then get space to reflect. We are then alone with our thoughts to question our happiness. Is life just there to function through? Or is it there to be grabbed?

As Elaine progressed on her journey, she began to explore other elements of the ten steps. She created loving boundaries, she reduced negativity, she embraced self-care, and she tried complementary therapies for the first time. Her over scheduling ways have calmed. As Elaine approached her fortieth birthday, she realised that her life was out of balance; stress should not be your go-to state. Her lunchtime walks around the industrial estate where she worked did not amount to the outdoor lifestyle she craved. Her time with her children was limited during the week, and the weekend was jam-packed full. She made the brave decision to take a break from her work and review her lifestyle. She removed the pressure she was putting on herself and took time to really get to know her own needs and wants.

Elaine embraced her time off, doing all the things she had longed to do and missed before: spending time with her children during the school holidays, going on walks in the forest, and climbing hills. Rather than going to the gym to solely build her strength, she discovered a place of stillness through her yoga practice that she previously didn't know existed.

Her love of nature and connecting to nature grew. She could use her time in nature to help feel more connected and balanced. She took part in a women's well-being trek in the Scottish Highlands. This slower pace allowed a connection to a happy place. Whilst on forest walks now, Elaine is more aware and mindful of the beauty around her, the simple things. She loves meditating in the forest, connecting with her breath, and allowing herself to feel grounded.

Meditation became a regular home practice. Elaine uses the grounding practices mentioned, from essential oils to getting barefoot.

Elaine has created a life where she can listen and pay attention to her children; she is more mindful in her daily life and has reduced her stress.

Be free, Elaine.

Meditation

Meditation for me is the ultimate grounding practice. It gets me out of my head and connects me fully with the present moment. Using a grounding meditation and really visualising it can help with this connection and balance. Meditations which use trees or mountains are great for assisting with grounding. Using a guided meditation is helpful when you're starting out to assist you in visualisation. You can access my grounding meditation on my website, www.spiritandsoul.me or on the Insight Timer App by searching Susi McWilliam.

Grounding Exercise 2: Download or listen to my grounding meditation and then make yourself comfortable. Take a moment for yourself, and take time to listen and relax.

Crystals

I adore crystals, and they are something that I use regularly now to support myself. I collected some in my younger days, as I love anything shiny and sparkly. These awesome creations of nature pack so much amazing strength and power. During my period of ill health, a friend and reiki healer gifted me some, and that's where my love of crystals was reignited.

I use crystals and gemstones to protect myself, reduce anxiety, increase confidence, improve loving relationships, and help keep me grounded. Here are some of my favourites and how to use them. As a point of interest, all the gemstones and crystals mentioned are associated with root chakra energy. As I went on to discover further in my journey, keeping our chakras balanced plays a key role in keeping us grounded and living our best life. Our root chakra is associated with keeping us grounded, rooted to the earth, safe, and secure. It governs our fight-or-flight response. If you suffer from panic attacks, you'll be fully aware of this bodily response to situations. This is the area you will look to balance and strengthen.

Tiger's eye: This wonderful brown and golden crystal has a beautiful depth. It's a hugely protective stone, one which has a beautiful strength and inspires courage. This stone is said to balance and clear emotions, so it's the perfect one for balancing and grounding. I use tiger's eye in tumble stone form (a little piece of the crystal), in jewellery, and I also have a little tiger's eye angel. In a metaphysical sense, tiger's eye grounds and centres; it can help deepen meditation practice and protects from negative energies (see Chapter 2, "The Good, the Bad, and the Ugly: Protecting Yourself from Negativity"). This is a grounding favourite for me.

Smoky quartz: This is a great starter crystal to own. It's fabulous for removing any negativity and clearing trapped emotions and negative thought patterns. When we're anxious, stressed, or worried, we are so susceptible to picking up the energy of others. This is great for removing any energies you have gathered that aren't supporting you. Smoky quartz neutralises any negative energies and vibrations, allowing you to feel lighter, clearer, and more connected. I use this in tumble stone form or in a larger crystal form. It's a great one to have in your kit.

Red carnelian: This red crystal can vary from orangey red to deep red. It's all about courage again. Fear is such a body depleter. Red carnelian can help support you and allow your courage and confidence to flourish. It's a great one for motivation and determination. So if you find you're struggling due to low mood or feeling that you can't take any more, this will help you through. I have a beautiful bracelet with these stones, but you could get it in whatever form works for you. It's a gorgeous one to use.

Clearing and Cleansing Your Crystals

Crystals absorb your negative energies, so it's important to cleanse them regularly. It's super simple to do and keeps them working at their highest vibration. I use various methods; here's some to get you started. You can hold your crystal under running water, visualising all the negative energy being washed down the drain. You can place them in a basin of salt; salt is a fabulous cleanser. Make sure you leave the crystals for a minimum of twenty-four hours, and then dispose of the salt. Don't reuse it. Next up, place your crystals outside in the moonlight (amazing to do on a full moon), and allow them to be cleansed and recharged using the moon's energy. Most of the time, I use white sage to cleanse my crystals (see Chapter 2 for more on white sage). You can buy a bunch and light it. Once lit, you hold a crystal within the smoke, allowing the sage to clear the crystals. White sage has a strong smell but is amazingly clearing for crystals. It's also good for yourself and your home. White sage is used as a cleanser in many cultures and has been shown by scientists to clear the air of bacteria and release positive ions, which are linked to mood improvement; triple-win: clear crystals, clear air, happier you.

Grounding Exercise 3: Picking and using your crystals can be super fun. If you have a local crystal shop, pay it a visit and pick some stones for yourself. There are lots of online crystal stores to pick from. Crystals hold so much support for you. Once you have selected your crystals, you're going to want to keep them close to you. If you're feeling stressed or worried, you can hold one in your hand and tune in; give it a little squeeze. Sleep with them under your pillow. But my favourite way, which always makes people chuckle, is popping them in my bra. Yep, you read right: pop it in your bra so it's close to you. Try to remember that they are there; when you go for a swim, shower, or the gym, there is every likelihood that they will fall and clunk on the floor. Always good for a laugh and embarrassed scramble. For the males amongst you, you can pop them in a trouser pocket and keep them close, anywhere that is close: on your desk, in a handbag, or in your wallet, so you can access them when you need to.

Bathing: As discussed in more detail in Chapter 9, "Flying Solo," taking an Epsom salt bath is hugely beneficial for the purposes of grounding you. They're a great way to balance your body and reduce negativity, connecting you back to earth. Don't have a bath? Try soaking your feet in a mix of Epsom salts and warm water to draw out impurities and connect you back with the earth.

Grounding Exercise 4: Fill your bathtub with water and between 250 and 500 grams of Epsom salts. I like the water pretty warm, as you will sitting in it for a while. Sit in the bathtub for around twenty minutes without using any other soaps or shampoos. Allow the magnesium to penetrate your body and ground you. So simple, so nice, and so powerful.

Grounding Food

We discuss food and nutrition in Chapter 4, "Feeding Freedom," but the foods we are discussing here are specifically for grounding. When you have that spacey feeling kicking in, head all over the place, this is where to start feeding yourself the right type of foods. Work out which foods you can eat to help ground you; it's easier than you think. Think foods from the earth, ones that have been grown underground and have soaked up lots of beautiful, nourishing nutrients from the soil. If possible, go organic to avoid adding additional toxins to your body, but if you don't have access to organic, then just wash your food thoroughly. Here's my go-to grounding list:

Ginger: This wonderful warming spice is great. I take ginger shots daily and I love adding fresh ginger root to teas smoothies and stir-fry. Available in most super markets now ginger is a fabulous one to reach for.

Root veg: carrots, turnips, parsnips, beets, and sweet potatoes. I love to make root veg soup: simple soups of just veg and stock, whizzed together to help nourish you, ground you, and comfort your body and soul. A great way to combine both above is to add to juices. Carrot, beetroot, and ginger are an awesome blend to ground and blast your body with nutrients.

Garlic: This little veggie is small but has huge health benefits. It's great to add to soups and hot dishes. This will not only help ground you; it will give you a mega immune-boosting hit at the same time to double-win. It's full of antioxidants and tastes amazing; pop it in your cooking and feel super connected.

Proteins: Eggs, beans, nuts, seeds, and meat are great for helping you feel grounded. When selecting proteins, decide what is best for you, what makes your body feel great. Choose organic, free-range, or grass-fed proteins, if possible. This will allow you to limit unnecessary hormones, avoid chemicals, and reduce any additional burden on your system.

Turmeric: Saving the best for last; I covered this golden beauty in Chapter 4, "Feeding Freedom." This is something I take daily. It comes from the same family as ginger; this root vegetable has a truly distinct colour. It is anti-inflammatory, reduces pain, and supports liver function. Taken in paste form, it can be made into a beautiful latte as a delicious way to incorporate it into your grounding ritual. It can be added to curry, stir-fry, or tea.

All the above are wonderful foods for feeding your root chakra, bringing it into balance, connecting you to the earth, and enabling you to feel truly connected, stable, balanced, and strong.

Grounding Exercise 5: Pick some of the grounding foods listed above and incorporate them into your diet this week. Make up a batch of soup for lunches; drink ginger tea instead of your coffee, and see how you feel. Go for it. You'll love it.

Essential Oils

These are my last grounding tools. I use them daily. I'm an essential oil geek. I lurve essential oils and the way they can shift your mood super quickly. But when it comes to grounding, these are such a great way to assist and support you. When selecting oils, always ensure you use therapeutic-grade oils. I personally use only certified therapeutic-grade oils. That way you can ensure the safety and purity of the oils. That in turn means they will work for you. Specifically for grounding, I like to use oils topically and aromatically.

What does this mean? Applying oils topically means you apply directly onto the skin and to a specific location. Always use a carrier oil to dilute down in case of any sensitivity; this is why using a pure grade oil is best. Topically for grounding, I apply oils to the base of my feet and at the very base of my spine to my root chakra. Aromatically, I like to pop a drop on my hands and take a deep inhale, apply to aroma jewellery, or pop in the diffuser at home. Here are my suggested oils to support your grounding:

Vetiver: This is the champion of grounding for me; its earthy smell instantly transports me to a woody area. I used this oil the day of my mother's funeral, and it was such a support. This is quite powerful one, and it's one I would reach for if I was feeling ungrounded. It's great to get you firmly rooted back into life. As a side note, I could not stand the smell of this initially; I applied it to the base of my spine. You don't need to love the smell. You just need to be open to the therapeutic benefits.

Frankincense: This is the king of oils and comes from the resin of the Boswellia tree. It's a great one to use when feeling overwhelmed. I apply this to the back of my neck or diffuse when I am feeling a bit unconnected and separated, and it then transports me back to a grounded and stable state.

Patchouli: This for many invokes the smell of incense and hippies. My first introduction to this oil was to help with anxiety. I bought this oil purely for its stabilising qualities, and it worked. This oil really connects you back into your physical body. It helps bring you back to a place of peace.

Arborvitae: The Tree of Life. The Latin name for this oil means "to sacrifice"; it's all about surrendering and allowing life to flow. This woody smell can guide you from scatterbrained to composed and calm. Applied to the soles of the feet or diffused, this oil can really build on connection. This is also a wonderful tool to release suffering.

White fir: I love diffusing this oil. It's fresh and just instantly connects me to trees and being in the forest. It's really calming and blends nicely with frankincense. This will really improve your focus and clear that foggy you feeling you get when you're ungrounded.

As you can see, most of these oils are from trees; their energies are firmly rooted in the earth and soil. Essential oils are a beautiful, natural, and powerful way to support and ground yourself.

Grounding Exercise 6: Pick one of the oils above and apply one drop, diluted with a carrier oil (I love coconut oil), to the soles of your feet daily for one week. See how much more connected you feel to the world around you.

You may not need all the exercises and tools above all the time, but you should turn to them when you're really feeling spacy and ungrounded. They'll guide you and plant you firmly back into your body, allowing you to live mindfully and enjoy the present moment.

NOTES PAGE

Chapter 6
Breathe: Because You Need To; Exercises for Everyday Living and Crisis

I breathe in peace and exhale calm.

My chest feels tight, and I gasp for air. My lips tingle, and my head feels light. I can't breathe, and it's terrifying. My first few panic attacks were horrific. I was 15 years old and had no idea what was going on. Once they started, they became a regular occurrence. They became my body's go-to response in times of stress, anxiety, and worry; many times, they came for no obvious reason.

My mum was obviously terrified as she took me to the doctor, hypnotherapist, and homeopathist. These all seemed to help for a short period of time, but then the problems would reoccur. I remember being embarrassed and locking myself in the toilet, crying my eyes out. This embarrassment led to me harming myself. I felt stupid and different and out of control. I would slap my head, punch my face, and even hit my head on things. Goodness knows how I didn't give myself a severe injury, but I never did (thankfully). I hated myself and my body. Being a teenager is challenging enough as it is, without randomly hyperventilating and bursting into tears.

My panic attacks carried on from age of 15 to the age of 35. As I got older, I knew when one was coming. I would feel it building and bubbling. I would find a private place and allow it to unfold. I had a brown paper bag I would carry (there was one in our first aid box for use at home). I would use this little brown bag to regulate my breath. This bag would move in and out so rapidly as I held it to my mouth, but it helped get my breathing back to an even level. Throughout the years, I learned various coping techniques, some more valuable than others.

Have you suffered a panic attack? Even if you haven't, all the exercises and information in this chapter will benefit you. Our breath is such a powerful focus to reduce stress, overcome anxiety, and shift our mood. It can switch us from our flight-or-fight response back to calm and serene.

Breathing is something we frequently take for granted, yet without it, we wouldn't be alive. A lot of meditation and mindfulness techniques focus around the breath. Being aware of our breath allows us to get out of our heads and connects our minds and bodies.

You cannot breathe deeply and worry at
the same time. Breathe. Let the worry go.
Breathe. Allow the love and intuition in.
—Sonia Choquette

What does our breath do? Breathing is an incredible process. It allows our body to take in oxygen, which is needed for most of our bodily functions, including digestion, thinking, and moving our muscles. This all connects to our brain, which monitors our oxygen and carbon dioxide levels. Our brain then adjusts our breathing to support our bodily function. All super smart. Our outbreath is our body's way of detoxing. The body uses our outbreath to clear itself of carbon dioxide.

Our breath is key to supporting our nervous system and responses to stress, agitation, and anxiety. Our body has two nervous system responses: the sympathetic and the parasympathetic. Our sympathetic nervous system is triggered when we're scared or anxious; it causes us to breathe faster, we sweat, and our palms get clammy. It's our fight-or-flight response. Our parasympathetic system is where our brain triggers our body to lower our heart rates, reduce our blood pressure, and calm our mind. This parasympathetic state is where we want to be. And the magical and amazing thing is, we can actually trick our brain into being calm, even if we don't feel it. How do we do this? By using our breath. We can slow our outbreath to send a signal via our vagus nerve to our brains to turn down our sympathetic response and turn up our parasympathetic response. Genius and a great mind body hack to help calm us instead of going into full-scale panic.

The breathing techniques below have all helped me find peace and reduce anxiety. They are another tool in my Be Free toolkit to turn to in times of need. My clients use these daily to support themselves, producing clearer minds and calmer bodies.

These should be done with your eyes closed; however, if you have issues with balance or don't feel comfortable, keep your eyes open. Gently allow your gaze to lower. The reason we close our eyes is to tune out any external distractions; it allows us to connect better internally.

Let's get started. You can find videos demonstrating all of these techniques on my YouTube channel.

Yogic Three-Part Breath (Dirga Pranayama)

The first breathing technique I ever learned was the Yogic Three-Part Breath. This is a panic attack saviour. It's relaxing, and I regularly use this when I'm feeling stressed or overwhelmed. This is my choice of breathing when I go to the dentist. This is a yoga class favourite and is often used at the start of classes to help you release the day and connect into the present moment. You might have already tried it. It's such a relaxing and comfortable way to breathe.

This breath helps you to connect with your full range of breathing, utilising your chest, ribs, and tummy. So often when we are super stressed, our breath is shallow, quick, and comes from the chest. This prevents our body from getting the full inhale of oxygen. You can do this breath seated or lying down. When first learning, I advise lying down so you can really begin to connect with the movements of your body and relax fully.

1. Find a comfortable place to sit or lie down where you will not be disturbed.
2. Gently close your eyes.
3. Begin to gently connect with your breath. Feel your breath travelling in through your nose; your chest gently rises and falls. Nothing controlled

at this point, just experiencing and feeling your breath.

4. Now place your hands on your tummy. Feel the breath deep in your tummy as you breathe in and out. Stay with the breath here for four or five breaths, exhaling each breath fully.

5. Move your hands up to your ribs now. Draw the breath up from the tummy and breathe in and out of the rib area. Feel your hands rise and fall. Feel them separate as you inhale and go back together as you exhale. Stay here breathing for four or five breaths, exhaling fully after each breath.

6. Now place your hands on your chest. Draw the breath up from the tummy, through the ribs, and into the chest area. Feel your chest expand on the inhale and contract on the exhale. Now you've got it. This stage is the three-part breath.

7. Breathe fully into your tummy, ribs, and chest, and then exhale fully, slowly, and steadily.

That is how this breathing technique is traditionally taught. What I have discovered through my teachings is that my clients actually prefer to do this in reverse. We have found that breathing into chest, then ribs, then tummy and then fully exhaling is more relaxing for us, and many find it easier. But you can try both ways and decide what is most comfortable for you. Practice this seated. You can use it on a train, on a plane, in bed, wherever you feel you need that extra moment of calm. It brings you out from your head and into your body.

All the breathing exercises are there to help you relax, not for you to feel more anxious, worried, or uncomfortable. Some you will love, but some you may not, and that is absolutely OK. It really is finding out about your personal toolkit and go-to favourites.

Counting Breaths

Counting to focus our mind while breathing is a mindfulness technique that has been readily adopted by Western society. The simplicity and effectiveness of breathing in this way makes it a great tool. Counting breaths can present itself in a number of different ways. When using either of these counting breaths, I find it really comforting, relaxing, and reassuring to place one hand on my heart and the other on my abdomen. It's almost like giving yourself a loving hug.

I learnt one of my favourite counting breath techniques whilst reading *The Miracle of Mindfulness* by Thich Nhat Hanh. This book describes breathing: "Your breath should be light, even, and flowing, like a thin stream of water running through the sand. Your breath should be very quiet, so quiet that a person sitting next to you cannot hear it. Your breathing should flow gracefully, like a river." Hanh teaches the following counting breath:

1. Breathe in, count one.
2. Exhale, count one.
3. Repeat inhaling, counting two, exhaling two.
4. Continue until you reach the count of ten.
5. Once you reach ten, repeat the cycle again, starting at number one.

This type of counting breath helps to focus the mind; it stops it from wandering off and being taken to our worries or to-do lists or wherever it wishes to travel. It keeps the breath even and calm and flowing steadily.

The next style of counting breath is where the exhale is longer than the inhale. The science behind this form of breathing exercise is that the longer outbreath triggers the vagus nerve to send a signal to the brain to turn up our parasympathetic nervous system, allowing us to feel calmer and more relaxed. This style of breathing allows the body to detox and eliminate carbon dioxide from the body. This supports the lungs and calms the body (this is the opposite of the short, sharp breaths we take when anxious).

1. Find a comfortable place to sit or lie down.
2. Gently close your eyes.
3. Gently place one hand on your abdomen and one on your heart.
4. Tune into your natural breath, feeling the sensations as it travels in and around your body; take a few moments here.
5. Begin by breathing in for three and exhaling six; continue breathing like this for a few minutes.
6. If the three and six breathing is easy, you can elongate to four and eight.
7. Only do what is comfortable. If we stress the body by attempting to really push the timings, the body has a stress response instead of the calming response we are looking for.

Square Breathing

As this name suggestions, this style of breathing is all about keeping the breath equal and even. Some people like this style of breathing, as they can also visualise a square as they breathe. It's a completely personal preference. Some clients do not enjoy retaining the breath in this style of breathing; if you find this is you, then please omit this part. This is something you can maybe work towards.

1. Find a comfortable place to sit or lie down.
2. Gently close your eyes.
3. As you breathe in for the count of four, visualise you are breathing along the top part of the square.
4. As you reach the next side of the square, you retain the breath for a count of four.
5. We then exhale along the base of the square for four.
6. Retain the breath for four along the last side of the square.

Many of my clients struggle with the length of the retention on the sides of the square. We can switch it up to a rectangle. We breathe in for four, retain for two, exhale for four, retain for two. So in theory, we've just shortened the sides a bit. You can choose; you can change it. Nothing is static.

Grounding Breaths

Of all the breathing techniques, this is the one I use the most. This will help you feel more secure, safe, and grounded. When anxiety hits, we often feel very disconnected and light-headed; sometimes, we feel like we're not even in our own bodies. We wander around, feeling completely spaced out; it can be quite unnerving. This breathing technique allows you to feel connected back into your body and also to the ground beneath your feet. If you suffer from vertigo or balance issues, this will really support you. It's a technique that has brought me great comfort and strength. I would use this style of breathing while seated or standing, as opposed to lying down.

1. You guessed it: find a comfortable place to sit or stand.
2. Gently close your eyes.
3. Connect with your breath as before, noting the natural movement within your body.
4. Once you are comfortable, begin to visualise drawing the breath up from ground beneath you, up the base of the spine.
5. Draw the breath all the way up the spine to the crown of your head.
6. On the exhale, visualise that breath travelling from the crown of the head all the way back down the spine and into the earth beneath.
7. Continue to breathe in this way, up and down, drawing the breath up from the ground beneath.

This is a wonderful technique to use outside, whilst barefoot. It really connects with the earth beneath you.

If you suffer from social anxiety, I have used this one a lot in those situations. You can do this standing in any situation, with eyes wide open. You can even use it if you're in a queue at the supermarket and find yourself getting overwhelmed. Really feel your feet connected to the ground beneath you, and as above, visualise breathing up and down the full length of your body. Draw the breath up from the ground beneath you and breathe it back down through the soles of your feet into the earth below. It's great for concerts and other crowded situations.

Alternate-Nostril Breathing (Nadi Shodana Pranayama)

This is the marmite of breathing techniques. It takes time, patience, and practice. You might be thinking, *Well, Susi, that doesn't sound ideal for when I'm freaking out, head whirring, and I can't get my breath.* And the answer is, you're right. This probably wouldn't be the first choice for mid–anxiety attack, but it's a really valuable one to learn. This breathing technique balances the mind. This is my favourite for when I'm feeling a bit overwhelmed or confused by life. The rhythm and pattern calm me and allow me to get lost in my breathing. It now leaves me feeling more centred and clearer, but that hasn't always been the case.

The first time I learnt this breathing technique, I thought it was the worst thing in the world. I had started a new yoga class, and it was my first or second time attending. My anxiety was at quite possibly the worst it had ever been. I had started yoga regularly again to help quell some of my anxious thoughts and feelings. As we began to learn this technique, I felt sick and dizzy, and panic set in. I wanted to run out of that class and flee for my life. I was reasoning with myself in my head, knowing if I fled, I would probably never go back. So I faked my way through the breathing. I pretended I was doing it and just willed the class to end as quickly as possible.

I'm not telling you this to scare you, as this breathing technique is far from scary and really valuable. I want you to know that I have been there; with practice and patience, not just this exercise but everything gets easier. So be gentle, and only do what's comfortable. Are you ready to find your Zen?

1. Find somewhere comfortable to sit.
2. With your right hand, fold in your top two fingers.
3. Move your right hand up towards your nose with your thumb beside your right nostril and your two fingers near your left.

4. These are going to be used to close and block nostrils as we go through the practice.

5. To begin, place your thumb against your right nostril, blocking and closing it; exhale fully out of your left nostril.

6. Inhale through the left nostril.

7. Use your small and ring fingers to close the nostril.

8. Now you have both nostrils closed and are retaining your breath for a moment.

9. Release your right nostril and exhale fully and slowly.

10. Inhale through the right nostril, deeply and slowly.

11. Block the right nostril with the thumb.

12. Retain the breath.

13. Release the left nostril and exhale.

14. You then begin the cycle again, breathing in left.

To begin with, it can seem a bit awkward or tricky to get into the flow, but once mastered, it brings clarity and supports those who are overwhelmed.

Exercise 1: Try each of these breathing techniques. Not all in one day, but just scattered throughout your week. Find which ones are currently easy for you. Play around with ones which are more challenging. Find one your currently resonate with and use it.

These practices will help support you and get you from those moments of sheer panic or stress into ones which are more manageable and allow you to feel safe. Learning to breathe correctly is one is the most valuable tools in your toolkit. The simple action of pausing and connecting with our breath can be all we need to help us make that shift and find our Zen.

> If you want to conquer the anxiety of life,
> live in the moment; live in the breath.
> —Amit Ray, *Om Chanting and Meditation*

Notes page

Chapter 7
Meditation and Mindfulness: Hushing the Chatter and Finding Peace

I meditate, and my soul and mind are filled with peace.

When your brain is full to brimming, it can seem like an impossible task to find calm, peace, and space. Meditation has been a saviour for me. In this chapter, we'll learn simple tips, techniques, and ways to implement meditation and mindfulness into your day-to-day life, switching up your thought processes, reducing anxiety, and allowing you to find the peace we all long for. We don't have to be Buddhist monks, in a cave, or on a hilltop away from society to learn to meditate. We can do this safely and comfortably from our own home.

My first experiences of meditation were the fifteen minutes at the end of a yoga class. I lay with eyes closed under a cosy blanket, trying not to snore, trying to follow my breath and the teacher's guided words. During this period, I had moments of complete surrender, but other times, I couldn't wait for it to finish so I could run off and do something else.

I dabbled in and out of meditation and mindfulness activities throughout my life, searching for this so-called inner peace and Zen. I learned various styles, traditions, and different teachers. Once I started this journey of searching, I discovered I was my own teacher; there wasn't just one style that I thought, *Yes, this is me; I'm only going to practice this way.* I discovered I loved them all. I loved how some styles challenged me, and some brought instant calm. I loved how different styles and types of meditation helped me at different times.

I believe meditation and mindfulness are suitable for people of all ages, from all walks of life, and from all religions. I've taught classes from nursery-aged children to adults well into retirement. It can truly benefit everyone. Anyone can learn to meditate.

Benefits of Meditation

Meditation now is so scientifically researched that it's a proven method of reducing stress, anxiety, and depression. I joke in class sometimes, saying, "Think of a condition, and meditation will improve it." I've listed below some of the benefits that meditation can bring.

But joke or no joke, the list is endless. Meditation to me is where healing can occur; we can be freed from internal chatter and external noise.

- improves sleep
- reduces pain
- lowers level of depression
- reduces symptoms of PTSD
- lowers anxiety levels
- boosts mood and improves outlook
- improves concentration
- lowers blood pressure
- lowers cortisol levels
- encourages self-awareness
- boosts creativity and inspiration
- overcomes addictions

Is Meditation for You?

"Meditation's not for me." "I'm too busy to meditate." "I don't have time to sit still, chanting for hours." "I can't do it." "My brain's too busy for meditation." I have heard it all, and I can honestly say, meditation is for you. It is for everyone. By the end of this chapter, if you haven't already tried meditation, I hope that you find something you like or are least willing to try, as the benefits are profound and life changing.

In 2014, as I lay in my bed, brain travelling at 100 miles an hour, negative thinking controlling my life, I grabbed my phone and searched YouTube for meditations for anxiety, meditations for healing, and meditations for stress. I would listen for hours. I would find peace, comfort, and solace in these moments and for some time to come. It was a safe space for me and one where the tightness in my chest left me. From that point, meditation became a daily practice for me.

Mindfulness is a buzzword that I am sure you've come across in your bid to be anxiety free. Mindfulness is a form of meditation. It is a practice you can bring into absolutely everything you do. Mindfulness keeps your thoughts in the present moment, instead of racing off like a freight train down a crazy winding track.

Christina Rodenbeck's *Meditation for Everyday Living* has a great definition of both meditation and mindfulness. She defines meditation as looking inward, blocking out our outside world, withdrawing, and focusing within. Mindfulness is the opposite; mindfulness requires us to expand our awareness and develop our inner observer. We notice surroundings and heighten our awareness. I believe we need to use both to be free from anxiety.

Meditation and mindfulness need to become part of our being and lifestyle, used consistently for optimum effect. I see so many people who join classes, feel better within themselves, but then stop practising. A crisis hits, and then they begin again. I call this crisis meditation. Yes, crisis meditation will make you feel good, but a regular practice will make you feel even better. Allow your mind to get used to being in a relaxed state; let yourself know you are safe, calm, and grounded. I don't know where I would be without my meditation practice. It has supported me through anxiety, depression, grief, loss, marriage difficulties, and living with active alcoholism. It provided a safe place, a place where peace existed when the chaos of life was too much to bear.

Where to begin? As I mentioned previously, I taught myself meditation from the internet and various sessions at the end of yoga classes. This journey led me to try different classes, attend different events, and train to become a meditation teacher. There are so many options to try; with the creation of apps such as Calm and Insight Timer (you can find me and some of my meditations there, search Susi McWilliam), you can access meditation support 24/7. You cannot get it wrong. You don't need to follow a set structure, be led by a guru, or spend vast amounts of money. You can teach yourself. However, should you wish to practice in a group session or develop your practice further, there are lots of meditations groups and classes for you to tap into.

When teaching a class, I always ask people to write down their motivation to start practicing. This will be what you need to return to when you can't be bothered, or on good days when you think you don't need it. Developing a practice will make a huge difference to your life.

Exercise 1: Grab a pretty journal and write down why you want to start meditation. For me, it would have been "I am looking to find peace and calm my negative thinking"; it could be to show up as a better mum, to stop your heart racing, to feel the tightness in your chest subside. Whatever your personal why is, write it down and tune into what you're looking to achieve from meditation.

Loving-Kindness

Now that you know why you want to start, let's begin. The first meditation I teach my students is the Buddhist Practice of Loving-Kindness (Metta Bhavana). *Metta* translated means "love, beautiful, nonromantic, compassionate love for another," and *bhavana* means "to cultivate or develop." This meditation can be quite emotive but is hugely powerful and beneficial. I love it, as the repetition of the phrases allows my mind to remain focused and prevents it from wandering off. This meditation follows a set simple structure. You can watch a video of this on my YouTube channel.

The key phrases we repeat are as follows.

May I be happy.
May I be well.
May I be safe.
May I be peaceful and at ease.

Then we do the same for others:

May you be happy.
May you be well.
May you be safe.
May you be peaceful and at ease.

Start by repeating the first set of phrases for yourself. As you repeat these phrases, allow loving feelings to flood your body. Visualise your heart centre being filled with loving light. I recommend doing this with your eyes closed, visualising an image of yourself, almost as if you were looking in a mirror. Imagine a light shining from your heart centre to the heart centre of your visualisation. Really feel into this process. Repeat the phrases above three times for yourself.

Then move forward and repeat the second group of phrases, visualising someone you love. As above, visualise them standing in front of you, shining loving energy, and truly meaning the phrases as you shine love and kindness from you to them. Repeat the phrases three times for this person.

Next, move on to someone neutral, maybe a colleague or neighbour or even someone from your local shop. Visualise them standing in front of you, shining light from your heart to theirs. Wish them happiness, wellness, safety, peace, and ease. As above, repeat the phrases three times.

Then bring to mind someone you have conflict or difficulty with. Follow the same phrases and practices. Visualise shining loving energy from your heart centre to theirs. Despite how challenging this may be, repeat the same phrases three times for this person. Side note here: This can prove difficult and sometimes emotional, and that is all OK. You will find that the more regularly you practice this particular meditation, thinking of this person, your relationship with this person will change. Your feelings towards them or uncomfortable situations will become less confrontational or upsetting. You begin to detach from your emotions. It's hugely powerful and really helpful. Use this for situations where you find it difficult having a face-to-face conversation. This can even be used for people who have passed on or are no longer in your life.

Lastly, bring everyone together: yourself, the person you love, the neutral person, the person you have conflict with, and anyone else you wish to add (animals, pets, other family members, and the greater community), and repeat three times.

This is an amazing meditation. I hope it brings you much comfort. As you go through it, try not to judge who comes to mind; just allow. When my mum was going through cancer, I thought of my best friend instead of my mum, and I thought, Susi, how cruel are you? Your mum needs that love and kindness, and you're sending it to Mary, or if I think of one child and not the other, or if I think of Stuart as the one I love and also the one I have conflict with; all of these are totally normal. Just take it that your subconscious knows what is needed.

With regards to how many times you repeat the phrases, I always suggest three. This is not essential, but I find it allows you to truly connect and gives you a better chance of visualising each person, instead of whizzing through the practice. I like to say the phrases out loud, as this allows my mind to stay focused. I'm less likely to disappear off to what I'm cooking for dinner or an email I forgot to reply to. Another thing you can do with this meditation is, use parts of it to focus on specific people. This is particularly useful when working through conflicts and difficulties.

Exercise 2: Try the Loving-Kindness Meditation. Find somewhere quiet for around ten minutes. Sit comfortably, with your back straight; spend a few moments tuning into your breath and then begin the practice as described. Enjoy. Spend a few moments at the end, sitting and enjoying being surrounded and held by this loving energy.

Guided Meditations

This is where a lot of people start out on their meditation journey; it's a meditation I love and find really relaxing. I typically don't teach these initially, as some people can't keep their minds focused on the guided journey. A guided meditation is like listening to a story. It takes you on a magical journey and is also wonderful for children. As adults, this type of meditation can initially be a little tricky. It depends on the nature of your job or how your mind works; some adults don't engage with the creative and imaginative side of their brains so much. These are wonderful for escaping if I am feeling ill; they also help me fall asleep.

The beauty of guided meditation is that you are told exactly what to do. You only need to get comfortable and allow your mind to follow the journey. This style of meditation is readily available for free via YouTube and apps such as Insight Timer. A google search of guided meditations will pull up many options.

Exercise 3: Visit YouTube or your search engine and type "guided meditation for anxiety." Make yourself comfortable, and listen to your chosen meditation. Enjoy this moment of peace. If your mind wanders, that's absolutely fine; just allow it to return back to the journey.

So Hum

This is my favourite daily practice. This particular meditation is a simple yet hugely effective meditation; it offers clarity, provides connectedness, and calms my mind. It can be done sitting up in bed upon waking or seated on the floor or yoga mat. So Hum is a mantra-based meditation (a mantra is a specific word or words that are repeated; the words are traditionally Sanskrit, a traditional Indian language). The words often don't correlate with English terms, and it's important to not get lost in the translation. When doing mantra-based meditation, it's about the sound and vibration these words create. Om is a great example of this and one you may be familiar with. The So Hum mantra is silent; we repeat it in our minds. Translated, it means "I am that," referring to the part of the universe where we are all interconnected. This practice is best done seated. I have heard of people doing this lying down, but I feel seated works best.

Once you are seated, allow a few moments to sit with your breath. Allow your eyes to gently close. Allow your breath to settle. As you sit, begin to imagine that as you inhale, you breathe in the word "So" from the base of your spine, drawing the breath up. Then as you exhale, breathe out the word "Hum" and visualise your breath travelling down your spine. You continue breathing in this way, repeating the mantra as you inhale and exhale. You can do this for as long as you like.

Exercise 4: Practice the So Hum meditation as described above for three to five minutes (set a timer, if that's easier). At the end of your meditation, whilst your eyes are still closed, ask yourself, "What do I need to know today?" Hold no judgement; just allow what comes. It may be something profound, or it could be something really simple, like "Drink more water." This is a daily practice I enjoy doing first thing in the morning. It's really beneficial for calming my thoughts before they go into overdrive.

Case Study: Diane. Diane is a 51-year-old mum of two. When she first came to see me, she was suffering from depression. Her depression had caused her to feel guilty for not doing enough and not being enough. The depression led to anxiety about the future; comfort eating became her support mechanism, and she had forgotten to make herself a priority. After taking antidepressants, Diane began to recover and returned back to herself. Fast forward to today, and the transformation is phenomenal.

Diane works full time and has two teenage children; she has a busy life and juggles work, life, and a holiday cabin that she owns. She felt her work-life balance was way off, and she needed a solution to calm her mind and bring her clarity.

She previously had difficulty controlling her emotions and was seeking greater self-control. She decided meditation was the route she wished to try.

Diane started meditation classes with me just over a year ago. During this time, I watched her grow and develop, and I recognise just how amazing she is. She has begun to set loving boundaries, protect herself from the negativity of others, and feel calmer in her work and her approach with her children.

Her life may not have got any easier, but her approach and awareness have completely changed. Meditation is really a catalyst for change. She realised through group classes that it was OK for her mind to wander and it was OK for her to spend time away from home, doing something for herself.

From living on the sofa whilst depressed, Diane now attends Pilates and yoga, runs twice a week, and even does body combat.

Self-care has now become a necessity. Previously, this wasn't even thought about; it wasn't part of her process. Diane now enjoys doing things that make her happy: craft projects, reading, making cakes for friends, and taking adult swimming classes to brush up her skills.

This to me is what the Be Free lifestyle is all about; it's about finding solutions that support you, implementing them, and then living your best life, despite your circumstances.

Be free, Diane.

Mindfulness

Mindfulness is being in the present moment, fully engaging in the here and now. The breathing techniques in the previous chapter are mindfulness practices, helping to guide us back into our bodies and into the now. For anxiety sufferers, mindfulness is a daily practice than can slow their fast-paced and overthinking minds.

It lovingly guides us back to reality. Any activity you do can be done mindfully. Reading a book, talking on the phone, meeting a friend for lunch, and even driving to work can all be mindful activities. In today's fast-paced world, we are encouraged to be mindless, to do more than one activity at a time. We are celebrated for our multitasking ability. Multitasking, however, does not lead to contentment and peace. When we multitask, it leads to frustration, spreading ourselves too thinly. Mindfulness is the opposite of this.

Have you ever been at work, typing, reading an email, listening to someone on the phone, and trying to think about something else at the same time? Craziness. How overwhelming and stressful is that? How would it be if you just finished typing the email, called the person back when you were finished, and only focused on one activity at a time? It's the same if you're a stay-at-home mum. You're rustling up dinner, whilst paying a bill online and trying to help your kids with their homework. You end up feeling completely pulled in all directions and don't feel that you are accomplishing anything to your best ability. Mindfulness takes discipline and training. We have become so accustomed to doing it all at speed; it feels unusual to slow down and focus on one task at a time.

This concentrated focus provides accomplishment;

we work better, more efficiently, and to a higher standard. You even become a better friend, partner, and spouse by listening and truly being there for each other.

Exercise 4: Pick something you do every day; it could be cleaning your teeth, having a cup of tea, walking to work, writing an email, or calling a friend. Do it mindfully, only focusing on that activity, engaging with your senses, tuning in, listening, feeling, and seeing all that is around you. It might feel a bit strange at first, but what you discover can be so beautiful. I remember walking down a path near my old house one day and suddenly noticing the sound of the birds, the smell of the leaves, and the buds on some bushes. This delighted me so much. Previously, I had walked this path completely blinkered to it all, blinkered to the beauty and life around me, as my brain was away somewhere else in the future, panicking about something that may never even occur.

Mindfulness really is an amazing gift to give yourself. The more you practice it, the easier it becomes, and the more your world expands.

The present moment is filled with joy and happiness. If you are attentive, you will see it.
—Thich Nhat Hanh

Guided Body Scan

This meditation is a wonderful evening meditation. It is very relaxing and a fabulous way to guide your body into a restful sleep. It's wonderful during periods of intense stress and worry. The first few times you do this style of meditation, it helps to have someone guiding you through it (or at least listening to it). From there on, once you have done it a few times, you can visualise it yourself. Work your way from the top of your body to the bottom, or vice versa. The body scan meditation below is taken from the NHS website. All versions of this meditation follow the same principles; you can be detailed or do a general scan, depending on how much time you have.

This guided body scan meditation is intended to help you enter a deep state of relaxation. It's best if you can manage to stay awake throughout the entire exercise. Don't try to relax; this will just create tension. What you'll be doing instead is becoming aware of each passing moment and just accepting what is happening within you, seeing it as it is. Let go of the tendency of wanting things to be different from how they are now, and allow things to be exactly as you find them. Just watch the activity of your mind, letting go of judgmental and critical thoughts when they arise, and just do what the exercise guides you to do as best you can.

Lie down in a warm and private place, dressed in loose and comfortable clothing, at a time when you will not be interrupted. Close your eyes, and let your arms lie alongside your body; let your feet fall away from each other, and slowly bring your attention to the fact that you are breathing. Don't try to control your breath in any way, but simply experience it as the air moves in and out of your body. Notice your abdomen and feel the sensations there, as your breath comes into your body and your abdomen gently expands. Then notice your belly deflate as the breath comes out of your body. Follow the rhythmic movement of each breath, the rising of your belly on the inbreath, and on each outbreath, just letting go. Let your body become heavy as it sinks a little bit deeper into relaxation. Just bring full attention to each breath in each moment. As you observe your breath, you may notice that it changes on its own accord. It may vary in speed, rhythm, or depth, and there may even be occasion when your breath seems to stop for a time. Whatever happens to your breathing, observe it without trying to cause or initiate any changes.

As you sit, feel the sensations of your body. Then notice what sounds and feelings, thoughts, and expectations are present. Allow them all to come and go, to rise and fall like the waves.

Allow yourself to become more and more still.

You may find that your attention drifts away from your breath, and you think about other things or hear some noises outside. Whenever you notice that you're not observing your breath, gently bring your attention back to your breathing. During the meditation, if you notice that you are focusing on some feeling or mood or expectation, treat this as you would any other thought, and gently bring your attention back to your breathing.

Bring your attention to your feet, becoming aware of whatever sensations are there. If you are registering a blank as you tune in, then just experience nothing. As you breathe in, imagine your breath moving all the way down to your feet, and then when you reach your feet, begin your outbreath, and let it move all the way up your body and out your nose. Breathe in from your nose and out from your feet. Become aware of the shins and calf muscles and the sensations in the lower legs, not just on the surface but right down into the bones, experiencing and accepting what you feel here and breathing into it, then breathing out from it. Then let go of your lower legs as you relax into the bed or mat. Move into the thighs, and if there's any tension, just noticing that. Breathe into and out from the thighs. Then let your thighs relax.

Shift your attention to your pelvis now, from one

hip to the other. Notice your contact with the bed or the mat, and the sensations of contact and of weight and whatever sensations (or lack of sensations) you are experiencing. Direct your breath down into your pelvis, breathing with the entirety of your pelvis. As you breathe out, move the breath back up through your body and out your nose, letting your pelvis soften and release all tension as you sink even deeper into a state of relaxed awareness and stillness. Be totally present in each moment. Be content to just be and to just be right here, as you are, right now.

Direct your attention now to your lower back and just experience your back as it is. Let your breath penetrate, and move into every part of your lower back on the inbreath. On the outbreath, just let any tension, any tightness, any holding on just flow out, as much as it will. Then let go of your lower back and move up into your upper back now. Just feel the sensations in your upper back. You may even feel your ribcage, in back as well as in front, expand on the inbreath. Let any tightness, fatigue, or discomfort in this part of your body dissolve and move out with the outbreath, as you let go and sink even deeper into stillness and relaxation.

And now, shift your attention to your belly again and experience the rising and falling of your belly as you breathe. Feel the movements of your diaphragm, that umbrella-like muscle that separates your belly from your chest. Experience the chest as it expands on the inbreath and deflates on the outbreath. If you can, tune into the rhythmic beating of your heart within your chest. If you can, feel it as well as your lungs expanding on either side of your heart. Just experience your chest and your belly, as you lie here: the muscles on the chest wall, the breasts, the front of your body. And now just let this region dissolve into relaxation as well.

Move your attention now to your fingertips and to both hands together; just become aware of the sensations now in the tips of your fingers and thumbs, where you may feel some pulsations from the blood flow, dampness, or warmth. Just feel your fingers and expand your awareness to include the palms of your hands and the backs of your hands and wrists. And here again, perhaps pick up the pulsations of the arteries in your wrists as the blood flows to and from your hands. Become aware of your forearms and elbows. Notice any and all sensations, regardless of what they are. Allow the field of your awareness to now include the upper arms, right up to your shoulders. Just experience your shoulders; if there's any tension, breathe into your shoulders and arms, and let that tension dissolve as you breathe out. Let go of the tension, and let go of your arms, all the way from your fingertips right through to your shoulders. As you sink even deeper into a state of relaxed awareness, just be present in each moment. Let go of whatever thoughts or impulses to move come up; just experience yourself in this moment.

And now focus your attention on your neck and throat; feel this part of your body, experiencing what it feels like when you swallow and when you breathe. And then let it go. Let it relax and dissolve in your mind's eye. Become aware of your face now. Focus on the jaw and the chin, just experiencing them as they are.

Become aware of your lips and your mouth. Become aware of your cheeks and your nose, feeling the breath as it moves in and out of your nostrils. Become aware of your eyes and the entire region around your eyes and eyelids. If there's any tension, let it leave as the breath leaves. And now the forehead and temple, letting it soften to let go of stored emotions. If you sense any emotion associated with tension or feelings in your face, just be aware of that. Breathe in, and let your face dissolve into relaxation and stillness. Now become aware of your ears and the top of your head. Now let your whole face and head relax. For now, just let it be as it is. Let it be still and neutral, relaxed and at peace.

Now let your breath move through your entire body in whatever way feels natural for you. Move through the entire length of your body. All of your muscles are in a deep state of relaxation. Your mind is simply aware of this energy, of this flow of breath. Experience your entire body breathing. Sink deeper and deeper into a state of stillness and deep relaxation. Allow yourself to feel whole, in touch with your essential self, in a realm of silence, of stillness, of peace. See that this stillness is in itself healing. Allow the world to be as it is, beyond your personal fears and concerns, beyond the tendencies of your mind to want everything to be a certain way. See yourself as complete right now, as you are, as totally awake right now.

As the exercise ends, bring your awareness back to your body again, feeling the whole of it. You may want to wiggle your toes and fingers. Allow this calmness and centredness to remain with you when you move. Congratulate yourself on having taken the time to nourish yourself in this way. This state of relaxation and clarity is accessible to you by simply paying attention to your breath in any moment, no matter what's happening in your day. Let your breath be a source of constant strength and energy for you.

Exercise 5: Follow the guided body scan above. Find a version online or via an app, and allow yourself this moment of tranquillity and rest.

Creating Your Own Meditation Space

This can be really fun and hugely beneficial. A cluttered space leads to a cluttered mind. You don't need to have a huge amount of space to create your own meditation area. It can simply be a corner of a room or even a small shelf. Looking out over a garden or into nature is lovely but not essential. Find a quiet spot within your own home. Sit on a nice chair, cushion, or yoga mat. It's also a good idea to have some things that are meaningful to you: a picture of your family, a beach scene, or something from nature, maybe a shell, a plant, or a piece of wood. Candles can offer a nice focus and smell. It's about creating somewhere lovely, just for you, your own mini Zen location. You can also use this as a space for quiet reflection, reading, journaling, and so on. But it's all yours. By creating familiar smells and a beautiful location, you are more likely to ease your body into a meditative state.

Exercise 6: Create a mini-sanctuary in your home. It could simply be tidying a corner and removing clothes from a chair, or you could devote a whole room to it. Have fun with it; find lovely pictures, candles, and cushions. Enjoy creating a space just for you.

Meditation Posture and Additional Information

There are lots of different styles and types of meditation, so if one doesn't resonate with you, another one will. It's about finding what is right for you. Whilst meditating, you may think about other things, and this is totally normal; your mind will drift. You have spent most of your life with your brain racing; it takes time to find that inner stillness, but it will start to appear more frequently the more you practice meditation.

When meditating, you don't need to sit crossed-legs in a full lotus position. The main thing is for you to be comfortable, so you are less likely to fidget. You want your back to be straight; if lying down or seated in a chair, keep your legs uncrossed. If sitting in a chair, your feet should be flat on the floor. You are looking to have your body relaxed, not forced into a position or holding any tension. Your spine should be nice and straight, with your chin gently tucked in. It's all just good posture, really, nothing forced or controlled, just nicely aligned. My favourite way to meditate is seated cross-legged on a pillow (although I like lying in bed too).

You can meditate at any time of day; I regularly meditate more than once a day, especially during a busy or overwhelming period. For me, morning meditation is always a must. I've discovered that meditating first thing allows me to calm my mind and sets me up for the day ahead. Meditating in the evening is a wonderful way to put your day into perspective and calm yourself before sleep. It's a personal preference, so play about with it, and see what you like best. Choose what you find most soothing and relaxing.

Meditation can allow us to explore our emotions and even find answers to questions we've been asking. It's a tool that gets us closer to who we truly are. Sometimes, difficult situations or emotions may arise from the past as we meditate. This is one of the wonders of meditation; many are not prepared for this. It allows us to see ourselves as we are. It really is a joyous journey, with nothing to fear. We are in a space where we can shed the layers we have built up around ourselves.

Being more mindful throughout your day and pulling yourself back to the present moment will soon become second nature. It all takes time but is a beautiful journey.

Notes page

Chapter 8
Move, Stretch, Play: Finding Your Flow

Exercise strengthens my body and
mind. I love moving daily.

Looking back and reading my diaries and blogs, this was my least favourite thing to think about doing. It filled me with fear. I just wanted to remain in the safety of my own home; most of the time, I didn't have the energy or inclination to get out there and get moving.

I used to love running, yoga, riding horses—all sorts of exercise, but when you're stressed, anxious or depressed, that was the last thing in my mind, even though I knew it would help. Here's the deal, though: You are an individual and will be at a different stage on your journey than anyone else. Maybe fitness and exercise is your thing, and you train for marathons, or maybe you can't even get out of bed. But rest assured, there will be something here to help you and inspire you. Moving, stretching, and playing will help you find yourself and your joy.

You may think embracing and bounding into a new fitness routine is the way to go about things, but slow down there, my sweet. When we are stressed or exhausted, our body is already under a lot of emotional pressure. Your adrenals may be close to or already experiencing burnout. Although we may think hopping into a body combat class will help us shift up our strength, it may actually put undue strain on your already weakened systems, and the high you experience during the class may hit you with a bump after.

This truly is a personal journey, and one you need to meet yourself where you are currently at, not where you think you should be.

Little, Often, and Build It Up

When I first set out, I did learn the hard way. I started by slowly walking round my garden, and then I built up to going for a walk round my street. At weekends or if I had assistance, I would go farther, with my mum or Stuart or a friend holding my arm. Then because I managed that and wanted to be fit, healthy, and "how I used to be," I embarked on my running again. Boom, then I had a painful injury. Not cool, and I was pooped.

The saying you have to walk before you run is so, so true.

Point to note here, and alarm bells should ring if you have this thought: I wanted to be how I used to be. We will all experience this at some point; this will be your biggest hurdle to overcome. Comparisons to how you once used to live can cripple you; it took me years to realise I was not that same person. It really upset me that I wasn't able to ride my horse and compete to the standard I wanted, or run a 10k or even play on the trampoline with my kids. You are you, regardless of this. Pushing yourself into situations you're uncomfortable with can actually put you back a step. I know, as I would regularly push myself way out of my comfort zone to prove a point. It's not healthy and left me feeling like I'd been hit by a bus.

I'm not saying don't push yourself or that you'll never be able to do what you loved in the past, but when you feel disheartened because you're not how you used to be, know that it's not a bad thing. You have evolved, and the stress, anxiety, and depression will change you. These experiences allow us to look truly deeply at our behaviours and actions; we can learn to change, develop, and grow them to support ourselves fully.

You are who you are now, not who you were years

ago, last week, or even yesterday. Every day offers the chance to grow and experience things we may have never considered.

Exercise is a fantastic tool to help raise our mood and vibe. It's a great way to boost our serotonin levels. Serotonin is an important chemical that helps regulate our mood, social behaviour, appetite, sleep, memory, and sexual desire and function. Winner.

One of the main reasons exercise is so important on this journey is to release tension. When we are anxious, we feel small; we contract our muscles when we feel fear or worried. Our posture changes, and then we transfer our emotional experiences into physical conditions and pain. All the exercises in this section will help you release those stress hormones and relax those tight muscles. You'll feel freedom and joy in your body again.

Let's get started with some ideas that can make moving, stretching, playing, shaking, running, and dancing all super cool; it's fun for all abilities.

Walking

Walking is a man's best medicine.
—Hippocrates

Whether it's around your house, in the garden, or a long walk through a forest, this is a magical place to start. You could maybe start by setting yourself a time or number of steps and build it up from there. I love being at the beach, so when I was able, I loved to walk. Being outside lets us connect again with the world. It creates a larger opportunity for us and allows us to escape from feeling trapped. Equally, this can sometimes cause a little fear, and this will happen. But breathe; take nice deep breaths as you go. When you return to your cosy chair or bed on your return, feel that sense of achievement and joy. Walking is a wonderful, low-impact form of exercise. A study at the University of Cambridge discovered that a twenty-minute walk a day cuts your risk of premature death by almost a third. How amazing is that? It also reduces your risk of stroke, heart attacks, Alzheimer's, and here's the key point for us: It is scientifically shown to naturally boost mood and lower stress.

Exercise 1: Find where you're comfortable just now. Set yourself a target or goal, maybe to walk to the end of your road and back. Or if you're feeling pretty fit and healthy, head to a woodland trail or the beach and go for a roam. Do this twice for the first week and build from there. Note down your activity in your journal so you can look back and monitor your progress. Step to it.

Case Study: Monika. Monika is a 37-year-old single mother from Croatia. When she first came to see me, she was experiencing stress, had anxiety, and was exhausted.

Today, it's a very different story. She is calmer, happier, more grounded, and feels more balanced. Her faith in God and love of spirituality have returned. I chose her as a case study for this chapter not because she's an all-out gym bunny, but because she is an example that wherever you are on your journey, any kind of movement is better than none. Monika had slept around twenty hours a day due to her depression; her brain was exhausted with overthinking and anxiety. She was trapped in a negative thought cycle. The four hours she was awake, she spent feeding her daughter and putting her to bed again. Her breath was quick, and she was living in survival (flight-or-fight) mode.

Monika now enjoys a number of activities, including walking in her local park, dancing with her daughter whilst she's cleaning, cutting the grass, singing, and engaging with her inner child in a playful way. She has also discovered kundalini yoga. But the main thing is, she has learnt to recognise and identify any symptoms that she is pushing herself too much. When this happens, she rests and sleeps and honours what her body needs. So movement doesn't need to be hitting the gym hard; it can be found in the simplest of tasks.

Monika has immersed herself and is still working through the ten steps. She has rediscovered her trust and love for God through meditation and deepening her spiritual side. She now looks after her body with self-care rituals, bathing, reading, and making alone time a priority. She's created boundaries from negativity and has realised it is not her responsibility to support or fix others. She loves mantras, breath work, essential oils, crystals, and reiki. She is on a journey of healing which is leading her to feeling empowered, more assertive, and in control yet calmer, happier, and more connected.

Be free, Monika.

Play

Sexual pleasure may be the last thing on your mind when you're stressed, in a low mood, and down. However, having an orgasm can actually help your body detox and raise your mood. It boosts endorphin levels, which flushes cortisol (stress hormone) out of the body, reduces inflammation, assists with getting a good night's sleep, boosts immunity, and increases levels of the hormone oxytocin, the hormone of bonding and love. After researching four thousand women, the *Journal of Psychosomatic Research in the US* discovered that people who orgasmed regularly were healthier and happier, had an overall higher quality of life, and had a more regular menstrual cycle. The beauty of this exercise is, you don't even have to leave your bed. You can do this flying solo or with your partner. Either way, you will benefit; if it's with your partner, I'm sure they will be thanking you too. You may be excited by this exercise or nervous, but once you get into it, I'm sure you'll reap the rewards.

Exercise 2: Find a space where you feel safe, are comfortable, and won't be disturbed. Light some candles if you like and play some soft music to help you unwind and relax. Make sure you're cosy, and get to know your body again. Be gentle and loving with yourself. If it helps, you can fantasise about your favourite crush; close your eyes and be in the moment. If you are with your partner, enjoy the connection you are feeling. Take it slow if you find it a little nervy, or take it fast if you're ready to go. Neither is right or wrong. It's about enjoying yourself, playing, having fun, and finding your happy spot. Gently bring yourself to arousal. If you wish, you can use stimulation such as a vibrator or toy;

it's entirely what you would like. This is about you. Be free, in the moment, and enjoy. Attempt this exercise once a week, and see how you begin to relax, shine, and radiate joy. Let's bring that sparkle back to those eyes.

Yoga

I adore yoga; it's one of my favourite ways to start the day and unwind. Yoga allows you to improve your posture, strengthen your core, and bring your body back into alignment. The spiritual journey yoga has taken me on has been a truly transformational one. I cannot rate starting a class highly enough.

There are so many types of yoga; whether you love the spiritual elements or are all about flexibility, there will be a class and style to suit you.

I started my yoga journey when I was a teenager, suffering from panic attacks. Mum took me to see this funny, round little lady. I would stifle my giggles as people would break wind, and she'd use words I'd never heard of. But looking back now, I'm so glad I was introduced to yoga and meditation at this point. I'm not the most flexible, and I can barely touch my toes, but all of that is irrelevant.

The success of yoga does not lie in the ability to perform the postures but in how it positively changes the way we live our life and our relationships.

—T K V Desikachar

The journey of self is more important than standing on your head. What you may find, though, is the actions you take on your mat will begin to affect your life. As you become stronger and more flexible on your mat, you will become stronger and more flexible in your attitude.

I'd dipped in and out of yoga; during my worst period of anxiety in my early thirties, I decided to jump in again. I'd been doing bits and pieces at home, but I was never sure if I was doing it right or holding myself correctly. So I booked to do some yoga classes. I went along to the class but was petrified. I learnt the breathing technique Nadi Shodhana. Translated, *Nadi* means "flow," and *Shodhana* means "purification." In the Western world, this is called alternate nostril breathing (this is discussed in chapter 6). The pace of my breathing was already through the roof, and my dizziness was horrendous, but this distraction and concentration eased my mind. I couldn't close my eyes and felt like I wanted to run out of the class, but I did it. I survived, and I keep going back for more.

Yoga offers so many benefits: It improves flexibility, builds strength, improves your posture, boosts immunity, reduces blood pressure, regulates your adrenal glands (lowering stress hormones), reduces anxiety (both mentally and physically), relaxes your system, helps sleep, and increases self-esteem. And that's just to start with. You seriously need this in your life (Timothy McCall, *The Yoga Journal*, 2007).

Exercise 3: Find yourself a yoga class and book a block. By booking the block, you'll be more inclined to be consistent with your practice. You can start this at home if you are unable to attend a class, although I highly advise you to find a class where a trained teacher can inspire and guide you, allowing you to discover how to perform and hold postures safely.

Running

This is one form of exercise where you will see results fast; it improves mood, strength, and sleep, and has been clinically shown to reduce depression. This is due to your brain pumping out feel-good chemicals such as endorphins and endocannabinoids. Running allows you to burn off that anxious energy; you can quite literally run from your problems. It clears the mind and allows greater clarity. Running isn't without its drawbacks, however; pressure on joints can lead to injury if not managed correctly. You can place undue stress on your already compromised body. So I would only advise running once you've built up to it. Start slowly, and enjoy the journey.

Running is the greatest metaphor for life,
because you get out of it what you put into it.
—Oprah Winfrey

With all these exercises, there are metaphors for life; you may struggle to begin with, but you will grow with strength and consistency.

Exercise 4: Grab your trainers; it's time to go. Start off slow, and build up. Base it totally on where you're at now. I suggest using a running app. It will allow you to track your progress; many them even have programmes you can use when starting out. I love getting outdoors to run. It's more interesting; you can connect with nature, and it's more varied. It's all a personal preference. There are also loads of running clubs available in most town and cities, offering support and friendship for all levels. Whether you start running for one minute or half an hour. Starting is key. Jog on, my lovely.

Shaking

I saved the best for last in this chapter. Who knew that dancing, shaking, and moving around like crazy could shift your mood up, release pain and trapped energy, and get those vibes high in no time? Seriously, this works. Even the smallest of movements, like shaking out your wrists or moving side to side; do whatever works for you. Do you sometimes feel like a ball of muddy energy? Anxiety, stress, and depression cause us to feel small, our muscles to contract, and residual energy to get stuck in our bodies. This leaves us with inflammation and pain and the feeling of being trapped.

I haven't gone completely nuts; this is actually a physiological response that can help the body reduce its own stress and restore balance and health. When animals experience the fight-or-flight response, they often follow this with muscle tremors. This is the body's natural way of soothing, settling, and releasing muscle tension caused by fear. The official name for treatments which trigger a tremor response is "trauma release exercises." This method is being used around the world to support victims of post-traumatic stress.

Reported benefits include less worry and anxiety, more energy, reduced muscular and back pain, increased flexibility, relief from chronic conditions, and fewer symptoms of post-traumatic stress.

When I started doing this, I never even knew this was an actual therapy. I just knew I needed to release the stagnant energy in me somehow. I would literally stand and shake and move and feel better.

The act of shaking gently bounces our organs and stimulates our lymphatic system. This allows our body to reduce unwanted toxins and waste from the body.

One example of this moving and shaking is Osho Dynamic Meditation; this an hour-long, powerful movement-based meditation to shift energetic blocks and break old ingrained patterns. This is a powerful and intense method of moving energy.

With all these movement ideas, there may be a sense of discomfort, feeling embarrassed, or fear. But push through, my lovely, as the other side of fear is joy.

> Life begins where fear ends.
> —Osho

You could take classes in therapeutic movement and dance, but the beauty is, you can boost your mood, increase your health, and have fun in your own living room. A study in the *Harvard Business Review* suggests that dancing reduces stress, improves mood and cognitive skills, and increases levels of the feel-good hormone serotonin. A study by the University of London states that dance can scientifically reduce anxiety.

Dance is about self-expression. Anything goes. The combination of movement and music can lift up your spirits.

Exercise 5: Grab your music and get ready to move, sway, shake, jiggle, and wriggle. Pick your favourite tunes and start. Don't try or force anything. This exercise is all about having fun, laughing, moving, and releasing all that anxiety. Allow it to flow out of your fingertips, release it into the air, and allow it to be free. If you like, you can sing, jump up and down, whatever works for you. Think 5-year-old's birthday party, and go for it. Wiggle your bottom; allow that tightness in your back, neck, and shoulders to slide away. Struggling for songs to play? Check out my "Shake, Dance, Play Playlist" on YouTube. Dance to your own rhythm, have fun, smile; you deserve it.

Psychology Today states that regardless of what form of physical activity you do, exerting yourself will cause the brain to release the mood-lifting neurotransmitters serotonin and norepinephrine. Plus, physical activities release endorphins, brain chemicals that promote euphoria and satisfaction. Exercise allows us to reduce the flight-or-fight response we experience during anxious periods.

I know how I felt after even the shortest of walks or wiggles. You got this. Allow yourself to move, stretch, and play. Find your flow, and be free.

Let's get this mood-boosting party started.

Notes page

CHAPTER 9
Flying Solo: Self-Care, Self-Love Rituals, and Routines to Support Your Healing

> My happiness is a priority; I completely
> love and accept myself.

So often when we are stressed, we get lost in a sea of people-pleasing. We lose our connection with ourselves, and this can make us fearful and anxious. Learning to love, nourish, and support ourselves is key to feeling connected, loved, and safe. Love will always overcome fear. There's some beautiful suggestions and exercises within this chapter to support your journey to self-love. This chapter will nourish your mind, body, and soul, bringing back joy and connection to self.

For most, self-care is viewed as a luxury or something to do after catching up on housework, putting the kids to bed, finishing that assignment, and the list goes on.

Our heads hurt with stress, but rather than deal with stress, we'll take a tablet; we're tired, so we'll have a caffeine-laden drink. Our skin breaks out, so we'll put make-up on to hide it. You're beginning to get the picture. In the Western world, we're very much about treating symptoms and quick fixes. We're always so busy carving out a life, making a living, that we fail to see the big picture.

If we do not have our health, we have nothing. We can't get to work, look after the kids, and care for loved ones.

This is how I came to discover reiki, meditation, and a more holistic life. My body eventually had enough. It was showing me so many red flags, giving me all the signs to take care. Yet I ignored them all. It then gave me the biggest signal of all: It decided to stop working. I was riddled with anxiety, panic, stress, poor diet, low energy, balance issues. It had given me many chances to take stock, but now, it was time for the biggy. Completely exhausted, down, and at rock bottom, I finally decided to listen.

So many people have this same story. It takes for us to be completely and utterly consumed with pain or run down to make the positive changes our body craves. People reach this point and feel like a failure, which is so far from the truth. The only failure has been failing to listen to our bodies and our hearts until it gets to a crisis point. So many of my clients come to me at this point.

I am aware that self-care isn't a luxury but a necessity. I learnt this the hard way, as so many do. The phrase "You can't pour from an empty cup" is so true.

In November 2016, I wrote a blog post titled "Self-Care Isn't Selfish." I said, "We must recognise our own needs as well as others. Life is not just about survival, but truly living, enjoying and embracing each day. When we look after ourselves it allows us to better cope with the challenges life throws at us. Circumstances will come and go and how we respond and react to these will be a direct reflection of how well we feel within ourselves. If we are responding from an already heightened level of stress the response will be very different from that of someone who is calmer and in a more balanced frame of mind."

Are you truly living, enjoying, and embracing each day? What are your current self-care rituals? Do you have anything in place just for you?

At my most anxiety-stricken, I would say there was probably zero time for me. I was flying around from one thing to the next, and even if I did do something which could be classed as self-care, I wasn't enjoying it or getting the benefit from it. My head and mind would be racing, already having rushed off into the future and panicking about something that hadn't even happened yet. I certainly wasn't experiencing self-love.

I was pushing my body and punishing it in some very unloving ways.

We're going to pare it right back, get back to basics, and get this self-loving journey off to a great start. Let's start with the basics.

Sleep

Did you know that sleep is a basic human need, not an added bonus? I say this half-jokingly, but actually, we all know this. But how many of us sacrifice sleep? I know I did (and occasionally, I still do). But as soon as I do, I feel it big time. The Surrey Sleep Research Centre states that up to 20 per cent of us suffer from some form of sleep disruption or disorder. It is suggested we need nine hours of sleep a night to function correctly and allow our bodies to heal appropriately, although this varies, dependant on age. The table below outlines recommendations from the National Sleep Foundation. This is a great starting point for assessing what the optimum and normal ranges are and will help you work out if you're getting enough sleep.

Age	Recommend Sleep	Might Be Suitable for Some But No Less Than This
Newborn	14–17 hours	11–13 hours
Infant 4–11 months	12–15 hours	10–11 hours
1–2 years	11–14 hours	9 hours
3–5 years	10–13 hours	8 hours
6–13 years	9–11 hours	7 hours
14–17 years	8–10 hours	7 hours
18–25 years	7–9 hours	6 hours
26–64	7–9 hours	6 hours
65+	7–8 hours	5 hours

Lack of sleep can play a huge role in contributing to symptoms of depression, anxiety, overeating, irritability, forgetfulness, lack of concentration, clumsiness, lowers your sex drive and is likely to increase your chances of an accident happening.

WebMD states, "Over time, lack of sleep and sleep disorders can contribute to the symptoms of depression. In a 2005 Sleep in America poll, people who were diagnosed with depression or anxiety were more likely to sleep less than six hours at night.

"The most common sleep disorder, insomnia, has the

strongest link to depression. In a 2007 study of 10,000 people, those with insomnia were five times as likely to develop depression as those without. In fact, insomnia is often one of the first symptoms of depression.

"Insomnia and depression feed on each other. Sleep loss often aggravates the symptoms of depression, and depression can make it more difficult to fall asleep. On the positive side, treating sleep problems can help depression and its symptoms, and vice versa."

Getting sleep is essential. How can we make sure were getting enough? How can we help ourselves get a great sleep?

I love using my fitbit app to monitor my sleep patterns. This was my main reason for getting one. It's so easy to think you're getting enough sleep and maybe going to bed early, but are you actually sleeping? Or are you surfing the web, watching a movie, reading, or scrolling social media?

It's time to get mindful over your bedtime routine. Here are my go-to tips for a fabulous night's sleep.

- Ensure you create a routine. Our bodies love routine, especially when it comes to sleep. Try to set a regular bedtime and wake up the same time each day.
- Work out what time you need to go to bed based on what time you need to get up. It's too late to

suddenly think I need eight hours sleep at 11.30 p.m. when you need to be up at 6 a.m.

- Make your bedroom a sanctuary, a beautiful and relaxing place to be, free from clutter.
- Reduce your caffeine intake later in the day.
- Try and get some daylight during the day. Leave the office at lunch or get some natural light. Artificial light really confuses our system.
- Reduce exposure to blue light items, such as laptops and mobile phones, prior to sleep.
- Use a diffuser and essential oils to help relax your system. Oils such as cedarwood and lavender are great supports.
- Have your bedroom at a relatively cool temperature.
- And lastly, clear your mind with some journaling or a gratitude practice to reflect on your day. Focus on the good, and use your breath to help calm your nervous system.

Exercise 1: Create an evening bedtime routine. Work out your optimum bedtime and wake-up time, and look to establish a beautiful, self-supporting, and nourishing sleep practice. Watch how your mood, clarity, and emotions increase positively.

If you are having consistent issues with sleep or

believe you may have insomnia, seek professional help. Book to see your doctor to rule out any other underlying conditions.

Food

Are you eating to nourish and support your body? Or are you eating to punish it? In Chapter 4, "Feeding Freedom," we look at food to support and reduce anxiety, but our attitude about food is also hugely important. Are you eating foods as an act of self-love? Yes, eat the cake, and enjoy and savour and delight at the wonder of the flavours and textures. It is only if we then beat ourselves up and berate ourselves that there is an issue with these kinds of treats.

My emotional issues with food began in my late teens and twenties. For me, this is an area I consciously and always have to work on, to identify why I am eating the way I am. Is it to block difficult emotions, pleasure, or punishment? All habitual responses take time to work through, especially emotional ones. So be gentle with yourself along the way. Look to your body as your friend. Look to support her, thank her, and provide her with the fuel to help you feel vibrant and glowing.

Values

Compromising your needs and values to help others is so counter-intuitive. Yes, you feel good initially when helping someone else, but if it's a continued thing and your values feel compromised, you will feel resentment. Resentment makes us feel like a victim and takes away our power. Not sure what your values and needs are? Values are moral principles and beliefs. My life coach and friend Calea Souter defines values as "who we are in our lives, right now, in this moment. Not who we'd like to be or think we should be. They stand for our unique essence, they are our most fulfilling form of relating and expressing. Values serve as a lighthouse guiding us to our true self. When we honour them, life is satisfying and blissfully abundant."

Making sure our values are honoured and fulfilled is an act of self-love and valuing ourselves.

I found that my key values are those of community, freedom, connection, accomplishment, honesty, integrity, independence, and service. These areas are the ones that drive my decision making; they are the ones that when fulfilled allow me to feel content. By ensuring that I do activities that fall into and meet my core needs and values, I feel happier, am more loved, and believe my life is fulfilling. Some other ideas of core values include family, healthy work-life balance, religious beliefs, loyalty, joy, trust, positivity, spirit of adventure, health, being ethical, dependability, respect, and passion.

Here are some examples of my core values, how I meet them, and what happens if I don't:

Connection: I love feeling connected to the people in my life, so maintaining this is key to my happiness. I love going on dates with my husband, catching up with friends for a cuppa, and FaceTiming my sister and family in Australia. When I allow this value to be compromised, I feel disconnected and a bit stressed; being totally honest, I find my heart aches and yearns for the feeling of connectedness.

Freedom: I never realised how important this was to me until my life got so busy and overwhelming that I no longer had it. Freedom for me is having moments where I have nothing in the diary or calendar, times when I can be spontaneous, times where I can do take myself for lunch, read a book, and just be with myself. Things that trod on this value include overscheduling, making myself too available to others, giving up my free time to do something someone else wants me to do. I need to schedule me time, the moments where I can walk in nature and just be. This is the time when my body feels relaxed and my heart says thank you for allowing me to be and for listening.

What you will find is, if someone does something to damage one of your core values, this will upset you. Honesty and integrity are important to me. If someone doesn't follow through on what they say they will do or hides something from me, this really upsets me.

Exercise 2: Let's work out what your values are; this exercise is so valuable. I worked through this exercise with my life coach, and it's something I return to, to this day. It will allow you to find out more about yourself, and once you recognise the things you love and value, you can then go about making them a priority. The other benefit is when you get upset or resentful, you can have a look and understand why. What value has been compromised?

Grab yourself a cuppa and journal, and really tune into what it is you value. Spend some time thinking about the things that are important to you, things that really bring you joy and help you feel fulfilled in life. Start with the things you love doing. What is it about these things you enjoy? Then you can look at things or people you don't enjoy or can't relate to. What is it about them that you dislike so much? This may lead you to a belief of yours that they are trampling on. Once you have written this down, you can begin to daw from this list what your values are and look at ways to honour them.

Now that you have a list of values, rank how you feel you're meeting them, 10 being "I am absolutely rocking it" and 0 being "I am doing nothing whatsoever to support this value." Let's now look at your lowest scoring value and decide if it's something that's truly important to you. If so, what can you do to raise this score? And how soon can you do so? The table below is a great way to stay accountable in meeting your values and needs. You can download copies of this core value tool by visiting www.spiritandsoul.me.

Core Value	Score	Actions to Increase Score	By When?
Connectedness	4	Schedule dinner with my girlfriends	15/01

Return to this activity monthly and keep track. Ensure you're keeping to and creating new value-supporting activities because you are important.

Self-Care Rituals and Routines

Adding and scheduling self-care into your daily and weekly schedule is often the only way it will happen. When working through a meditation class on self-love, I asked my clients what self-care was to them. Here are some of their current rituals and routines:

- taking a bath
- running
- meditating
- reading
- sleeping
- cooking a nutritious meal
- having time to yourself
- taking yourself on a lunch date
- coconut oil pulling
- yoga
- massage
- going for a walk in nature
- listening to music
- buying yourself flowers

I'm going to highlight a couple of these. Many of the list above will be covered throughout the book, and I'm sure you can think of a few of your own to add to this list.

Bathing

I ask clients of my Be Free Anxiety Programme to do this twice a week. Not just a beautiful bubble bath, but an Epsom salt bath. Epsom salts are salt crystal that produce magnesium when dissolved in your bath. This has been a solution for muscle aches and pains for hundreds of years. But the benefits of this type of bath are much more than for muscle aches and pains.

Magnesium is a key mineral required by our bodies to function efficiently. It supports a huge number of bodily functions, our cells, and our nervous system. It is anti-inflammatory and can be used to support our bodies in reducing stress responses. Magnesium is used by the body during periods of stress. Deficiencies in magnesium are linked to depression, headaches, migraines, chronic fatigue, insomnia, and many other symptoms and ailments. Many of us are deficient in this key mineral.

In Dr Josh Axe's article "9 Signs You Have Magnesium Deficiency and How to Treat It," he discusses the main causes of magnesium deficiency: soil depletion, GMOs, stress (both emotional and work stress), digestive diseases, and chronic disease. He also discusses the symptoms, which can include cramps, insomnia, muscle pain, anxiety, high blood pressure, diabetes, fatigue, migraines, and osteoporosis.

For our health, the three key areas are anxiety, fatigue, and insomnia. Magnesium supports our central nervous system, and by supplementing magnesium, we are assisting our body in calming and reducing stress.

Exercise 3: You guessed it: Time to get those Epsom salts out. When Epsom salts are dissolved in water, they are absorbed through the skin and replenish the level of magnesium in the body. The magnesium then helps to produce serotonin, a mood-elevating chemical within the brain that creates a feeling of calm and relaxation.

For full benefit, you need to bathe in the salty water for twenty minutes before using any soap or shampoo. Start with around 250 grams of salts per bath. Grab some salts, find a good book, and soak yourself happy.

Don't have a bath? Then grab a basin and can do exactly the same by soaking your feet. I recommend you do this twice weekly.

Coconut Oil Pulling

My best friend introduced me to this many years ago. As a coconut oil lover and being game to try anything that could improve my health, I gave it a go.

Oil pulling is a traditional Ayurvedic technique used

for detoxing in your mouth. It has been used for centuries as a traditional Indian remedy for numerous conditions, including tooth decay, bad breath, whitening the teeth, boosting the immune system, strengthening the jaw and teeth, and the biggy for me: reducing inflammation and toxins throughout the body.

How does it work? As we sleep, bacteria and toxins build within the mouth. Oil pulling is done first thing in the morning prior to eating, drinking, or brushing. The oil pulling works by cleansing and detoxing the oral cavity. It sucks and draws out all the nasties. The antiseptic and antibacterial coconut oil cleans up your mouth.

You take a spoonful of coconut oil or an oil pulling tab. You can make these yourself at home. Simply melt some coconut oil in a jug or bowl. Pour whilst runny into an ice cube tray and allow to set (I like to add three drops of therapeutic-grade peppermint essential oil to my mix). I pop these into a pretty Kilner jar by my bedside so I can grab one first thing on waking. But to start with, I literally had a jar of coconut oil and a teaspoon by my bed and would scoop it straight into my mouth.

Once you have your oil, let the fun commence. At first, it will be quite unusual. I think it's a marmite activity; some people love it, and some not so much. Once you get past the unusualness and tune into the results, it's amazing. Pop your oil in your mouth; if solid, it will begin to melt. Then it's time to engage your inner child and swoosh it around your mouth and through your teeth, as if it were jelly. Pull the oil in and around your mouth. Continue to do this for around fifteen minutes. You can wander around doing yoga, meditating, showering, or prepping for your day ahead. Once finished, you want to spit the oil directly into the trash (not your sink).

Small activities like this can be built into your day, making your health and your mind a priority. These are acts of self-love.

Me Time

Creating a date day for yourself is such a wonderful act of self-love and self-care. It doesn't need to be a whole day. Just taking yourself out for a cuppa at a coffee shop with a few stolen moments and great book is a wonderful way to let yourself know that you matter. I love scheduling these moments and find them so necessary. These moments, I feel free. Anxiety and stress can make your world feel small and overbearing. When we create these areas where we are entirely free to pick and choose what we do, that is when the anxiety releases, and we get a true sense of what it is to be calm and joyful.

Exercise 4: Time to take yourself on a date. It can anywhere and for however long you can create. Take a notebook or journal with you. Spend some time journaling what you can do for self-care. Create a list you can turn to when you're feeling the stress and anxiety build. Build it into your daily, weekly, and monthly routine. This can be super fun. Just allow it to flow, without judgement. Have fun.

Once your cup is overflowing, there's plenty time and energy to share. You show up as the best version of yourself. It's a win-win. It's time to show yourself love in all areas: the food you eat, the words you speak, the actions you take, and how you move and love your body.

Notes page

Chapter 10
Dare to Be Different: Complementary Medicine and Alternative Therapies.

I love trying new things and welcome
new ways of thinking.

What started off as a cry for help and feeling like there were no other options led me to discover some amazing and natural solutions to support my journey. In this chapter, we'll discuss the benefits of different forms of healing therapies, why try complementary medicine, and why they are such an awesome way to support your path to feeling amazing. They ultimately led me to my calling in life and my career as a holistic therapist and coach.

The benefits of alternative therapies are vast. Recent studies from the University of Minnesota suggest that half of all those with anxiety or depression try some form of alternative treatment or holistic therapy to help cope with symptoms.

I remember lying in bed, after having a meeting with a neurologist. I wasn't getting any answers to why my body felt so bad. Everything felt out of balance. I had a fleeting thought back to trying to conceive and how I had gone for acupuncture sessions to align by body's hormones. I made a call and booked in for a session. I showed the Chinese doctor my tongue and described how I was feeling; she told me I was suffering from extreme stress. She applied the needles and left me in a candlelit room whilst they worked their magic. After she removed them, she gave me a really vigorous massage around my neck and shoulders. When I left the clinic, I felt more balanced, both mentally and physically.

Acupuncture

Acupuncture is a form of traditional Chinese medicine. Needles are applied to pressure points and meridian lines (energy lines) to balance qi, which is our energy within our bodies. It is believed that when this energy is blocked or imbalanced, it can lead to pain, discomfort, and disease. The energy is balanced by placing very fine needles into the skin to create a flow of energy within the body. Although a form of complementary medicine, acupuncture is now carried out in many mainstream clinics and also available via the NHS. Your session normally begins with a very through consultation. During this time, the doctor assesses your needs. Acupuncture is a treatment which balances your whole body; even if you go for one reason or symptom, you find other symptoms improve. It is designed to bring equilibrium into your being.

The Centre for Integrative Medicine in San Diego and also the British Acupuncture Council have many links showing the clinical and scientific evidence of acupuncture in supporting a huge range of conditions, including chronic pain, migraines, anxiety, depression, cancer symptoms, hypertension, hormonal imbalance, PMT, menopause, allergies, muscular pain, and nausea. When selecting a practitioner, I highly recommend looking for someone who is associated with an official registered body to ensure they have the appropriate level of training and expertise in their field.

Reiki Healing

A few years later, I was yet again in bed due to severe vertigo and anxiety; my best friend suggested I try reiki. I had no idea what is was or what was going to happen. I visited the house of a woman my friend recommended, with no expectation or indeed understanding, just my best friend telling me I needed to try it. I chatted to the practitioner prior to getting up on the couch; I cried and sobbed as I explained how I was feeling. I was then asked to lay on the couch. I was anxious and worried, and in my head, I remember thinking, *This isn't going to work.* I lay there for around forty minutes, and when it was finished, I felt a little spaced out but felt lighter and more confident. This was the start of my reiki journey. As I drove away that day, something had changed in me, and I knew this was the start of my reiki love affair.

Reiki (pronounced "ray kee") is a Japanese form of energy healing. Like acupuncture, reiki is used to identify and address any imbalances in energy within the body. The word *reiki* means "universal life force." The practitioner channels this life force energy and transfers it to your body. Developed by Buddhist Mikao Usai in 1920, it recognised that we could take responsibility for our own healing by utilising this universal energy, coupled with the reiki principles of "Do not anger," "Do not worry," "Be grateful," "Work honestly," and "Be kind to all living things." It's extremely loving and safe. Due to the fact it doesn't involve any manipulation of the body, this treatment is suitable for all ages and conditions. Reiki stimulates the body's own healing processes. It works mentally, physically, emotionally, and spiritually. Reiki can be used to shift old patterns and beliefs, reduce physical pain, and ease stress, depression, and anxiety. To me, it's like lovingly guiding you home.

> Reiki is love, love is wholeness, wholeness
> is balance, balance is wellbeing, wellbeing
> is freedom from disease.
> —Mikao Usai

When receiving a treatment, you are fully clothed and either lying down or seated. Practitioners will hover their hands above you and feel for any imbalances. They will then move and work in specific areas, rebalancing and aligning the energy. Some people will experience heat, tingling, or coolness; some people see colours or drift off to sleep. Each person and each session is different. I highly recommend it as a support to your overall mental and physical well-being. I go and visit my practitioner once every six weeks and use reiki as a support between sessions.

Aromatherapy and Essential Oils

Essential oils are a wonderful natural support, Mother Nature's healers. Essential oils come from the leaves, stems, bark, flowers, and skins of plants. They are what gives the plant its natural aroma. If you have ever smelt a rose, the leaves of a mint plant, or the rind of a lemon, you have smelt essential oils. Essential oils can be used to support our bodies and minds physically, mentally, emotionally, and spiritually.

Essential oils work fast and extremely well within our bodies and brains; this is due to them being natural, so our body knows what to do with them, unlike synthetic products. The molecules are so small that they can cross our blood-brain barrier and get into our systems quickly. The effectiveness of essential oils varies drastically, depending on the quality. Quality of essential oils varies, depending on where they have been produced and how they have been distilled. So finding the best quality and most natural oil is recommended. I use only therapeutic-grade oils to ensure that they have no fillers or synthetics added.

In 2017, the Tisserand Institute did a systematic review of twelve clinical trials looking at aromatherapy as a tool to support depression. "The review concluded that aromatherapy shows potential as an effective therapeutic option for the relief of depressive symptoms." In 2013, the Department of Pharmacology, Institute of Biosciences in São Paulo, Brazil, studied the effect of citrus oils for supporting anxiety and depression and showed that bitter orange essential oil can boost serotonin levels, improve our mood, and lower anxiety, stress, and depression. The study of essential oils is developing at a rapid rate as more and more people seek natural options and solutions.

My study and research of essential oils started in 2015. Mum had developed terminal cancer, and I was seeking any form of natural solution to support her mentally, physically, and emotionally. The more I learned, the more I reached for them myself. I used them to support my stepson's autism and improve his focus and concentration; it helped my family's immune system, as I was so concerned my mum would catch something. I turned to them myself for emotional support during a challenging and extremely difficult two-year period. Essential oils as a support tool blew my mind; they worked fast, and their effectiveness was amazing. I then began to use essential oils with my clients, and it all grew from there. I am continuously learning new uses, and new studies are being carried out. It's something that has been used for thousands of years, yet currently, it's an area that is experiencing huge growth in the support of mental and physical health.

There are three ways you can use essential oils: aromatically, topically, and internally. Internal usage is only suitable with certain oils, and the oils must be labelled as such. Internal usage is only suitable for therapeutic-grade oils; many shop-bought oils are not that pure. The early stages of my essential oil journey was very reactionary; I mostly used it for physical ailments, coughs, colds, burns, that type of thing. Now the majority of my essential oil usage is proactive support for my body. I use them a lot to support my emotional health. I have created my own essential oil protocol to support clients dealing with anxiety which you can find further details of at my website.

Essential oils work very quickly to support your emotions, especially when used aromatically. They can bring your body into a state of balance. When inhaling essential oils, the oils directly enter the olfactory system and then lead to the limbic system in our brain. The limbic system has glands that support our mood and emotional responses. This is a super quick way that we can take control of our emotions before our emotions take control of us.

Amanda Porter's book *Emotions and Essential Oils: A Modern Resource for Healing* explains why essential oils can support our emotional health: "As the oils secure our physical health, they provide us with the energy needed to penetrate the heart and enter the emotional realm. Essential oils raise the vibration of the physical body. As the body lives in higher vibrations, lower energies (such as suppressed emotions) become unbearable. The body wants to release these feelings. Stagnant anger, sadness, grief, judgment and low self-worth cannot exist in the environment of balance and peace which essential oils help to create."

Below, I've outlined my main go-to oils to support various moods, emotions, and conditions you may experience. I advise you to inhale these oils directly from the bottle, or pop a drop on your palms and take a deep breath, or apply to the back of the head at the base of your skull. Always ensure the oils you are using are therapeutic-grade oils. You can find further support regarding this at my website or work alongside an essential oil professional.

My Top Five Anxiety Oils

Wild orange essential oil, as mentioned in the studies above, is a go-to mood-boosting and anxiety-quelling oil. The smell will transport you to sunny climbs and lift your mood and spirit. This is a great double-whammy oil, increasing positive emotions and reducing worry.

Lavender essential oil is one you may be familiar with. Often associated with peaceful sleep, lavender can be used to calm and relax the body. It allows the body to be more peaceful whilst increasing our ability to express our emotions in a positive way.

I was given bergamot essential oil by a friend during a period of low mood. I would apply a drop to the base of my nose, and it helped me feel more confident and calmer. It's often used for its antidepressant qualities.

Lemon essential oil has an unmistakable smell. It is one of my favourites and one I use daily. This essential oil is commonly used to support anxiety, depression, and grief, to boost energy, and to uplift mood.

Frankincense essential oil is a wonderful oil that helps you to feel calm, grounded, and connected. This oil really triggered my study of essential oils. This oil is wonderful in supporting the body on a cellular level; it eases symptoms of depression and assists with emotional balance. It's great for mental fatigue and overall nourishing of the body mentally, physically, and emotionally.

Everyone is an individual; essential oils may work differently with different people, based on their chemical make-up. The suggestions based above are common uses for these oils.

Massage

When we are stressed, anxious, or depressed, we often carry ourselves differently; our posture is compromised, we curl our shoulders, and we feel small. Tension and stress build within the body, which can then lead to pain and discomfort. The phrase "carrying the weight of the world on your shoulders" is quite true. I know when I feel anxiety creeping in the first place, I feel it in my shoulders, followed by my lower back. For many of my clients, it's in their neck, which often leads to migraines and tension headaches.

> Massage is not just for the physical body, but the emotional body too. Touch can often trigger and release emotions such as grief, anger and anxiety within a safe environment. The therapist carries a responsibility to ensure the client is comfortable and at ease. Trust is an essential part of the healing process.
> —Erika Cowie, massage specialist (luckily for me, my bestie and massage guru)

Releasing the tension within our bodies through massage is a great way to release the build-up of stress and emotion. Massage comes from a wide range of cultures and backgrounds; there are so many different types to try. There really is something for everyone. Massage can be done seated or lying down, clothed or unclothed. Massage works by manipulating the body's muscles and tissues. It releases tension and toxins, improves circulation, reduces pain, and balances stress hormones. Massage can bring about a state of relaxation, offering our bodies the opportunity to find moments to heal and recharge.

Massages vary in levels of pressure that's applied; some use essential oils, such as aromatherapy massage. You could try Swedish, hot stone, deep tissue, reflexology, and shiatsu massage. Massage is a deeply personal choice; find what brings you the most relief and relaxation.

Exercise 1: Pick some form of alternative treatment and give it a try. Schedule some self-care and healing into your schedule. You and your body deserve this chance to heal and balance.

Alternative therapies are expensive, will vary from culture to culture, and have been used for hundreds of years. What I adore about looking at alternative therapies is that they are all encompassing. They look to bring balance to all the systems in the whole body: hormones, mental, physical, and emotional. Harmony is what our body is seeking; I love this quote by Edward Bach:

The medical school of the future will not particularly interest itself in the ultimate results and products of disease, nor will it pay so much attention to actual physical lesions, or administer drugs and chemicals merely for the sake of palliating our symptoms, but knowing the true cause of sickness and aware that the obvious physical results are merely secondary, it will concentrate its efforts upon bringing about that harmony between body, mind and soul which results in the relief and cure of disease.

—Dr Edward Bach

Notes page

Chapter 11
What Now? Moving Forward and How to Sustain Your Best Life

Every day is a blessing; I love my life.

You've read the book; you've done the exercises. What now? Now is the time to turn all the good you have done, all the work you have put in, to create a lifestyle of joy, freedom, and happiness. This is the exciting part; you are more than capable of implementing change. Living a lifestyle free from anxiety, depression, and stress is so simple in principle, yet so many of us struggle with it. By making loving decisions and creating a schedule that supports us, mind, body, and soul, we can be free.

I want you to succeed. You deserve to feel that tightness leave your body, your mind to slow, and tap into how it feels to find peace. In order to achieve this, we need structure, routine, and loving habits. This will allow us to build consistency into our days and success into our lives.

Success doesn't come from what you do occasionally;
it comes from what you do consistently.
—Marie Forleo

Every day is an opportunity for a fresh start, to try something new. As you move forward with your life, be gentle yet passionate in your approach to creating a lifestyle that supports you. Depression and anxiety are never far away and will wait to pop back when they can. It's our responsibility to keep this from happening.

How can we limit depression and anxiety? Only by embracing a new lifestyle that supports and sustains our mental, physical, emotional, and spiritual health. You now have knowledge of the ten key areas I consider essential in living a life filled with freedom and joy. It's time to tackle these areas, one by one.

Life will consistently throw us curveballs, and just when we think we've got it sussed, something else will get thrown our way. Whilst writing this book, I experienced some of the most painful experiences of my life: the death of my mother, the mental breakdown of my husband, and ongoing support to my family, husband, and self. Through all of this, there was stress and moments of complete shock and anxiety. Yet I did not break and crumble. The tools I have shared throughout the book and the exercises you have done are what kept me sane. This is a lifestyle that will support you through it all. Creating daily practices of meditation, breathing, and gratitude kept me from falling into panic attacks and despair.

I truly speak from experience when I say you can find relief naturally. When life throws us these challenges, we just need to reach for these tools. Eat well, make sleep a priority, and focus on the good around (however small that glimmer of good may feel).

Exercise 1: Take time to journal how you would like your day to look and how you would like to feel. Get deep. Really focus on all the things you would like in your life, not what you don't want. Get really clear. Once you've written this all down, take a moment to close your eyes and really visualise yourself as you wish to be: free, calm, and confident.

Tapping into how we want our life to be, getting clear on our thoughts, goals, and feelings, allows the magic to occur. It brings us closer to creating and manifesting the most amazing life.

Exercise 2: We looked at scheduling in previous chapters; now, it's time to schedule your best life. Grab a pen and paper or download my daily planner sheet, and let's work out how you are going to schedule your day for success. This is going to support you in creating your best life. What daily actions will you schedule to support your health? It's time to plan those support tools into your life. When will you wake, meditate, drink water, make dinner, see friends, read positive and inspiring words, plan your following day, and exercise? Whilst doing this, you will come up against resistance, I'm sure; it's new, but you get to design how your day looks. Leave windows for moments of freedom.

There will be days when your schedule doesn't go to plan and you just want to hide in bed. Be gentle, but step by step, inch by inch, your small lifestyle choices become habits, and then it will be second nature. Small, consistent, supportive decisions will have you feeling amazing.

On the days when you are feeling anxiety creeping in or you can't see the light for the darkness, nourish your body and mind. Take a moment to review the Be Free Anxiety Matrix and check on where you are in each of the areas (you can download our check-in sheet from www.spiritandsoul.me). This will help you identify where the stress, low mood, and anxiety are coming from. You'll begin to see patterns. So maybe you aren't making enough time for self-care, or you are saying yes to too many things. It takes time to change our conditioning and previous habits. As you go through each day, celebrate how far you've come. Write it in your journal, and review where you were before. Acknowledge your progress. When we are in thick of things, it's easy to overlook how well we are actually doing. Checking in with your mood, emotions, and overall health will allow you to see what wonderful changes you are making.

I can't wait to hear your success story and see you creating a lifestyle of joy, freedom, and happiness for good. Sending you love, hope, and a whole lot of courage.

It's your turn to be free.

Love,
Susi
xxx

Notes page

CHAPTER 12
Helpful Links and Support to Keep You Flying Free.

These are great pages and inspiring links to follow to support your journey to being anxiety free. People often ask me to suggest one book to help or wonder where I find support. This is the place to find the answers when you want to delve deeper.

First stop: www.spiritandsoul.me. Here you will find links to all the free downloads, tools, and support materials mentioned within the book. You can also find me on Facebook and Instagram at susimcwilliamspiritandsoul. On YouTube and Pinterest, you will find me at Spirit and Soul, Aberdeen.

What you consume via website, book, and podcast is really personal. What you resonate with, someone else may not. The key to picking a resource to support you is choosing something uplifting and inspiring. You can pick something educational, but your focus is something that leaves you feeling lighter and more empowered.

Supportive Books

The first two books are books that changed my life. The first book I recommend to all my clients and is one I regularly still delve into. This book is *You Can Heal Your Life.* To me, it's the bible of overcoming anxiety, and it really was a trigger for my own healing. The second book is *Light Is the New Black,* and this helped guide me back to myself and finding what I really wanted to do with my life.

You Can Heal Your Life, Louise Hay (Hay House, 1984).

Light Is the New Black, Rebecca Campbell (Hay House, 2015).

The Five Side Effects of Kindness, David R Hamilton (Hay House, 2017).

Calm, Fearne Cotton (Orion Spring, 2017).

Uplifting Prayers to Light Your Way, Sonia Choquette (Hay House, 2015).

The Tapping Solution, Nick Ortner (Hay House, 2013).

The Miracle of Mindfulness, Thich Nhat Hanh (Rider, 1991).

Blogs

My first blog where I shared my path to recovery: susimcwilliamthedizzybrunette.weebly.com.

Other blogs of mine are available at www. spiritandsoul.me.

Supportive Podcasts

The Anxiety Coaches Podcast

Rise Podcast with Rachel Hollis

The Calmer You Podcast with Chloe Brotheridge

Hay House Radio Podcast

Rise Together

Supportive Websites

www.spiritandsoul.me

www.mindful.org

www.mindbodygreen.com

https://tinybuddah.com

www.louisehay.com/

Apps

Insight Timer Meditation App

Calm

Headspace

Notes page

About the Author

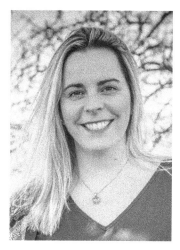

Susi McWilliam is a Meditation coach, Reiki practitioner and Speaker, founder of Spirit and Soul, training private and corporate clients in holistic approaches to supporting mental health.

Susi's friendly nature and modern day approaches to creating a life of calm and peace attract clients, and allows those who come into contact with her to leave feeling empowered and uplifted.

Susi was drawn to healing through her own life experiences. Having suffered from anxiety and then depression from her teens. Susi went through life struggling with anxiety and low mood for almost 2 decades. She spent most of this time researching and seeking solutions After finding freedom, and healing. Susi then went on further to study so that she could share her experience with others.

Susi owns The Sanctuary, Health, Wellbeing and Creative space in Scotland offering a range of workshops, classes and holistic treatments.

Her goal is to share and empower others to find solutions to their anxiety, stress and ill health using the bodies innate power to heal naturally.

Lightning Source UK Ltd.
Milton Keynes UK
UKHW011816171219
355552UK00001B/20/P